Electromagnetic Radiation Survival Guide - Step by Step Solutions

Including 5G and up to date EMF Info

expanded 3rd edition – 2021

Dr. Jonathan Halpern, PhD

Copyright © 2013 Jonathan Halpern

Cover design by: Jonathan Halpern and Karen Snashall

All rights reserved

ASIN : B00HKMCQEY

ISBN: 979-8596671865

ISBN-13: 978-1499323023

ISBN-10: 1499323026

Without limiting the rights under copyright reserved above, no part of this publication may be reproduced, stored in or introduced into a retrieval system, or transmitted in any form or by any means (electronic, mechanical, photocopying, recording, scanning, or otherwise), without the prior written permission of the copyright owner of this book. The scanning, duplication and distribution of this book via the Internet, or via any other means without permission of the author is illegal and punishable by law. Please purchase only authorized electronic or printed editions, and do not participate in or encourage electronic piracy. The characters and events portrayed in this book are fictitious. Any similarity to real persons, living or dead, is coincidental and not intended by the author.

DEDICATION

In memory of Dr. Wilson Wan, Ciril Kunstelj and Karen Snashall

ACKNOWLEDGMENT

I would like to acknowledge the late Karen Snashall for her help with cover design and Mr. S. Geri for his help with some of the photos.

CONTENTS

FOREWORD

"If we continue to develop our technology without wisdom or prudence, our servant may prove to be our executioner".

General Omar Nelson Bradley, former Chairman of the US Joint Chiefs of Staff

INTRODUCTION

This is the 3rd edition of the 'Electromagnetic Radiation Survival Guide'. Radio Frequency (RF) technology and the EMF and EMR it produces are evolving rapidly. We need to constantly keep up to date with recent developments in order to protect ourselves effectively against these health hazards. In the 3rd edition I've added a chapter dedicated to 5G and a section discussing 5G protection strategies. I hope to keep updating this publication with new developments in the Ebook version and in future paperback editions.

Jonathan Halpern, PhD

 21 January, 2021

PREFACE

I first became aware of the adverse effects that Electromagnetic Radiation (EMR) has on health when I got my first cell phone. Some may still remember earlier mobile phones models. Mine was rather bulky, had big buttons and a stubby antenna protruding from the top. After making my first phone call I felt a slight pressure headache but did not give it much thought. The headache dissipated after a few minutes but came back again following my second phone call. The pattern kept repeating itself consistently until after about a week I finally made the connection between using my cell phone and the headaches that also kept becoming more severe. That is how I first discovered that I was Electro-Hypersensitive (EHS) long before I knew the syndrome actually existed. In those days mentioning my "mobile phone allergy" to most people was not a good idea because it was usually received with raised eyebrows and skepticism. In a way I was lucky because at the very body told me that I need to be cautious. Ever since then, I have only been using my mobile phone in emergencies and have not been using Wi-Fi at home. On rare occasions when I am forced to use my cell phone, I get a headache often coupled with nausea. This repeats itself without fail even if I use the phone on speaker phone mode and to a lesser extent if I use an air tube headset. The severity and duration of the headaches are dose dependent: In other words, they depend on how long I talk on the phone and how close the phone is to my head. My electro-hypersensitivity triggered a keen interest in the body's electromagnetic fields and their role in health and disease. My research over the years has made me realize that many aspects of plant, animal and human life depend on a fine balance between positive and negative electrical charges, fine-tuned subtle electromagnetic fields and a constant electromagnetic flow on the cellular, tissue and systemic levels. The proliferation of electrical power and wireless technology is responsible for an exponential increase in electromagnetic fields (EMF) in our environment. The direct and unavoidable consequence is a massive and unprecedented increase in electromagnetic radiation (EMR) exposure. There is now substantial science backed and extremely disturbing evidence that EMR exposure has become one of the greatest health hazards of our time.

In 2011 The Parliamentary Assembly Council of Europe released a resolution on the potential dangers of electromagnetic fields and their effect on the environment. The resolution states that: *'Telecommunications and mobile telephony appear to have more or less potentially harmful, non-thermal, biological effects on plants, insects and animals as well as the human body, even when exposed to levels that are below the official threshold values'* [1].

The 2012 Bioinitiative report, the most comprehensive independent report to date on the effects of EMFs on health, states that: *'bio-effects of EMF are clearly established'* by well over 1800 independent studies[2].

It may take some time for the full consequences of exposure to various electromagnetic fields to become widely accepted by the scientific community, government and industry. Unfortunately, by that time many people may develop serious health disorders that will impact personal life and public health. I believe that for anyone who is serious about maintaining or regaining his/her health and the health of loved ones the time to deal with Electromagnetic Radiation (EMR) is NOW.

Dr. Jonathan Halpern, PhD (Health Sciences), MSc (TCM), BSc (Engineering)

21 January, 2021

DISCLAIMER AND LEGAL NOTICES

This publication is not designed to, and does not provide medical, technical or legal advice. All content ("content"), including text, graphics, images and information available on or through this publication are for general informational purposes only. While every attempt has been made to verify the information provided in this publication, neither the author nor the publisher assume any responsibility for errors, inaccuracies or omissions.

Any slights of individuals or organizations are unintentional. Any reference to any person or business whether living or dead is purely coincidental. If advice concerning medical, technical, legal or related matters is needed, the services of a fully qualified professional should be sought. The content is not intended for use as a source of technical, medical or legal advice.

The content is not intended to be a substitute for professional medical, technical or legal advice, diagnosis or treatment, testing, measurement, analysis or design. Never disregard professional medical, technical or legal advice, or delay in seeking it, because of something you have read on or through this publication. Never rely on information available on or through this publication in place of seeking professional medical, technical or legal advice. The writer and publisher of this publication are not responsible or liable for any advice, course of treatment, diagnosis, analysis or any other information, services or products that you obtain through this publication. You are encouraged to confer with your doctor and technical and legal experts with regard to information contained on or through this publication. After reading information available on or through this publication, you are encouraged to review the information carefully with your professional health care provider, legal and technical professionals.

You should be aware of any laws, which govern medical, legal and technical practices in your country and state The information presented herein only represents the view of the author at the date of publication.

Because of the rapid rate with which various conditions change, the author reserves the right to alter, modify and update his opinion and the content of this publication in accordance with the new conditions as he perceives them.

GLOSSARY

1G, 2G, 3G, 4G, 5G - 5 generations of mobile networks (G - stands for generation)

Beamforming - a method for directional transmission and reception to/from a specific device using combinations of antennas within an antenna array.

LTE - *'Long Term Evolution'*. A standard for wireless data transmission implemented since 4G

MIMO - *'multiple input & multiple output'* method for increasing radio link capacity using combination of multiple antennas

MMW - Millimeter waves - radio waves in the EHF band with wavelengths of 1 -10 millimeter

EMF – Electromagnetic Field

EMR- Electromagnetic Radiation

EHS – Electro-Hypersensitivity

Hz – Hertz (cycles per second)

KHz – Kilohertz (1000 cycles/sec)

MHz – Megahertz (Million cycles/sec)

GHz – GigaHertz (Billion cycles/sec)

ELF – Extremely Low Frequency

HF – High Frequency

LF – Low Frequency

VHF – Very High Frequency

UHF – Ultra High Frequency

SHF- Super High Frequency

EHF - Extremely High Frequency

RF- Radio Frequency

RFR – Radio Frequency Radiation

GS – Graham Stetzer

mG – Milligauss

DECT a standard for "Digital Enhanced Cordless Telecommunications," used in indoor wireless phone systems to connect the cordless phone to the base station that is connected to the phone line (landline).

1. ELECTRO-HYPERSENSITIVITY (EHS)

Are you Electromagnetic Hypersensitive (EHS)?

What is EHS?

Electromagnetic HyperSensitivity (EHS) also called Electromagnetic Sensitivity, electro-hypersensitivity, electro-sensitivity, electrical sensitivity (ES) and "Idiopathic environmental intolerance attributed to electromagnetic fields (IEI-EMF)". Based on a 2005 study the World Health Organization (WHO) concluded that:

"EHS is characterized by a variety of non-specific symptoms that differ from individual to individual. The symptoms are certainly real and can vary widely in their severity. Whatever its cause, EHS can be a disabling problem for the affected individual. EHS has no clear diagnostic criteria and there is no scientific basis to link EHS symptoms to EMF exposure. Further, EHS is not a medical diagnosis, nor is it clear that it represents a single medical problem." [3]

EHS is a new syndrome. Apparently it can be caused by the presence of electromagnetic radiation well below the "EMF Thermal Effect Threshold" safety standard set in the 1960's. This standard does not take into account well established bio-effects well below the "Thermal Effect" as described in the 2012 Bioinitiative Report.

EHS Symptoms

EHS may manifest in a wide and often confusing range of symptoms including:

1. Headaches that get progressively worse

2. Eye strain, dry eyes, blurred vision

3. Facial flushing

4. Tinnitus (ringing and buzzing in the ears)

5. Nausea

6. Dizziness

7. Shortness of breath, pressure in the chest

8. Irregular heartbeat

9. Chronic fatigue and weakness

10. Muscle aches and pains, fibromyalgia, arthritic pains

11. Prickling sensations

12. Numbness in fingers

13. Burning sensations

14. Skin rashes, itchiness, blotchiness or even whole-body skin symptoms

15. Stress, depression, anxiety, poor concentration, other mood disorders

16. Brain fog, memory loss, memory deficits confusion, disorientation

17. Disturbed sleep

CAUTION: Any of the above symptoms may also be associated with a wide range of other health disorders, some serious or even life endangering. If you experience any of these symptoms you need to seek the advice of a qualified medical practitioner for diagnosis and treatment.

Generally, EHS can be classified as mild, moderate or severe depending on the severity of the symptoms, their duration and their impact on the person's quality of life and ability to function in daily life. Mild EHS may manifest with mild symptoms such as prickling or burning sensations that disappear within seconds or minutes after EMF exposure (e.g. using a cell-phone) has stopped. With moderate EHS the severity, frequency and duration of the symptoms increase. For example, a headache may persist for several hours after using the cell-phone. With severe EHS the problem becomes chronic and persistent. A combination of symptoms described above may manifest with increasing levels of severity. For example, the person may develop chronic debilitating headaches and chronic fatigue. The person's ability to function in daily life is compromised significantly.

With time EHS symptoms tend to become chronic and often debilitating. Studies conducted in 2001 and 2002 revealed that people reported symptoms most frequently due to exposure to cell phone base stations (74%), cell phones (36%), cordless (DECT) phones (29%) and power lines (27%) visual displays and fluorescent lighting (1.9%), electrical factors and also chemicals or smells (2.4%)[4].

Electromagnetic hypersensitivity is not yet accepted as a medical diagnosis. Yet the number of people complaining of debilitating symptoms associated with exposure to cell phone base stations, cell phones, microwave towers, smart meters and other EMF sources is rising exponentially. Epidemiological studies on EHS conducted between 2001 and 2007 found prevalence of EHS to be 1.5% (Sweden), 3% (US), 4% (UK), and 5% (Switzerland). A 2002 Swedish study reported that 10% sufferers of EHS were either on sick leave or have chosen to take early retirement or were on a disability pension, compared to only 5% in the general population[5]. Clearly, regardless of the exact causation mechanism of EHS these are very significant findings.

Some scientists have referred to EHS as an allergic reaction to electromagnetic radiation. I think this is not such a good definition for several reasons. Although environmental and food related allergic reactions and EHS share some common symptoms they do not share the same chain of causation. The body's responses to allergens have been studied extensively and a range of allergens have been identified. This is not the case with EMF. So far numerous studies have shown that EMF exposure may result in a range of morbid bio-effects even at low levels and these effects may take place in totally asymptomatic individuals (i.e. people that do not display any symptoms or reactions whatsoever). The 2012 Bioinitiative report cites 1800 studies reporting a wide range of morbid bio-effects of Electromagnetic radiation (EMR) at much lower levels than the existing safety standards. These effects are subtle but cumulative. The bio-effects, described in these studies, include various forms of damage on the cellular and tissue level that do not lead to an allergic reaction. Although it is not always understood why some people become allergic to eggs whereas most of the population can eat eggs without having any problem, the fact remains that allergy to eggs is an individual problem and there is nothing inherently wrong with eggs. On the other hand, as the 2012 Bioinitiative Report points out - EMF may cause a range of morbid bio-effects in any individual regardless of the presence or lack of symptoms. This is where the biggest problem lies when making any analogy between EHS and allergic reactions. People who do not experience any reaction or symptom resulting from exposure to EMF may come to the wrong conclusion - that they personally do not have a problem with EMF and therefore they do not need to take the necessary precautions.

I believe that EMF should be treated as a form of an environmental toxin such as asbestos, mercury, cadmium, lead, BPA or radioactive particles. All of these toxins are present in the environment in varying concentrations and all are bad for us. They may trigger neurotoxic, genetic or carcinogenic effects. As their concentrations in the air, water and soil increase - so do their morbid effects. I believe EMF should also be treated as an environmental toxin and therefore, we all need to reduce our EMF/EMR exposure as much as possible.

People suffering from EHS should not be treated simply as unfortunate individuals who cannot enjoy the benefits of wireless technology and electrical power like the rest. They should be treated as the "canary in the coal mine" serving as an early warning for the rest of humanity. For those not familiar with the term "canary in the coal mine" - it originated when miners used to take caged canaries down to the coal mines with them. They positioned the cages on the ground. If dangerous gases (e.g. methane or carbon monoxide) leaked into the mine tunnels, these gases would cause the death of the canaries serving as a warning signal to exit the mine tunnels immediately. The morbid bio-effects of EMF described in the 2012 Bio-initiative Report may trigger a range of disorders including neurological conditions, infertility, birth defects and cancer. Many of these conditions develop slowly and silently over many years while the person is not presenting with any symptoms or complaints. And that is why we should treat the Electro-Hypersensitivity (EHS) syndrome and EHS sufferers - as a stark warning, alarm bells and sirens going off, that we should all heed to even if we still cannot see or feel the fire (yet).

2. ELECTROMAGNETIC FIELDS (EMF) & ELECTROMAGNETIC RADIATION (EMR)

Sources and types of Electromagnetic Fields

In order to deal effectively with EMF and the EMR it creates, it is important to understand how they are created and where they are coming from. Getting a good grasp of the basic concepts is important because different types of EMF/EMR require different protection strategies and measures. You don't need to be an engineer or a scientist to understand this section. It is written using basic terms and simple language.

The most common sources of EMF are:

1. Electricity in general, power lines, transformers and electrical appliances generate low frequency (**LF**) electromagnetic radiation.

2. Wireless technologies including cell phones, DECT phones, Bluetooth enabled devices, Wi-Fi routers, Wi-Fi enabled devices such as tablets and laptops, cell phone towers, microwave communication towers, microwave ovens and radars are responsible for rapidly increasing levels of radio frequency (**RF**) electromagnetic radiation (**RFR**).

3. Another source of EMF is called **"Dirty Electricity"** – a general term given for electrical currents contaminated by micro-surges - spikes that have superimposed themselves on top of the "clean" alternating electrical current (AC).

Table 2.1 Types of EMF

Types of EMF	
Earth's Magentic Field	Schumann resonance (approx.) 7.83 Hz / 14 Hz / 20 Hz / 26 Hz / 33 Hz / 45 Hz
Low frequency (LF)	**Extremely low frequency (ELF) - 3 Hz to 3Kz** **Very low frequency (VLF) - 3 KHz to 30 KHz**
Radio frequency (RF)	Very High frequency (VHF) 30 MHz - 300 MHz Ultra High frequency (UHF) 300 MHz - 3 GHz Super High frequency (SHF) 3 GHz - 300 GHz
EMF from Dirty Electricity	2 kHz to about 120 kHz

Electromagnetic Wave Frequency

EMF are differentiated and categorized according to their frequency and wavelength. The frequency indicates the number of times a wave oscillates per second and is measured by Hertz units (Hz). Please remember the following units as they will be used frequently in subsequent sections.

- One **Hz** represents **one** oscillation per second.
- One **KHz** represents a **thousand** oscillations per second.
- One **MHz** represents a **million** oscillations per second.
- One **GHz** represents a **billion** oscillations per second.

Electromagnetic Wavelength

The naked eye cannot see electromagnetic waves. They can only be viewed on a special device called an oscilloscope. The waves we deal with in this book mostly resemble a sine wave. A single wave cycle looks like this: The wave starts from zero, goes up, reaches a maximum positive peak, goes back down to zero, continues going down and reaches a negative trough and then goes back to zero. While going up and down the wave also propagates forward at the speed of light. The distance the wave travels forward during a single cycle is called one wavelength. The wavelength is inversely proportional to the frequency. In other words, the higher the frequency the shorter the wavelength; and vice versa - the lower the frequency the longer the wavelength. Typically, Extremely Low Frequencies (ELF) have wavelengths that can be kilometers long, whereas microwave Radio Frequencies (RF) of cell phone and cell phone towers are several centimeters long. This difference between the wavelength of ELF and RF is very important because it affects our ability to block and shield these waves.

Low Frequency (LF) Electromagnetic Radiation

Low frequency (LF) electromagnetic band is often defined as radio frequencies from 3 Hz to 30 KHz (there are other definitions but let's stay with this one). Within the LF band it is worth mentioning two sub bands – ELF and VLF defined as follows:

- **Extremely low frequency (ELF)** - 3 Hz to 3Kz
- **Very low frequency (VLF)** - 3 KHz to 30 KHz

In this book we will mostly be dealing with ELF. Specifically, in frequencies of electromagnetic fields associated with electricity (i.e. hi voltage power lines, power boxes, electrical wiring) and electrical appliances powered by Alternating Currents (AC) that are either 50 Hz or 60 Hz, depending on the country you live in, and also with their harmonics. Harmonic frequencies are complex waveforms that may be created as a result of using various electrical devices such as rectifiers and are often multipliers of the original frequency.

As the name implies electromagnetic fields have two components – an electric field and a magnetic field. To assess ELF, we usually measure the strength of the magnetic field component. LF meters are often only capable of measuring magnetic fields. The strength of the magnetic field is measured using two types of units – Milligauss **(mG)** units and micro-Tesla **(µT)** units. Milligauss is used more often than micro-Tesla. The conversion between the units is very simple and done as follows:

- **1 Tesla** = 10,000 Gauss.
- **1 microTesla** = 10 Milligauss

Low Frequency waves have very long wavelengths that can be several kilometers long. Due to their very long wavelength LF waves can diffract over and under obstacles and are extremely difficult to block or shield. This is the reason why the best strategy and often the only strategy to deal with very strong ELF radiation sources is avoidance, or put more simply – getting out of harm's way. One important example: To stay EMF safe we should avoid living or working in close proximity to high voltage power cables and pylons as they generate enormous levels of electromagnetic radiation.

Low level ELF radiation can be found everywhere. It radiates from fuse boxes (power boxes), electrical wiring, electrical transformers and rectifiers and of course from all electrical devices. The good news is that low level ELF radiation levels drop very rapidly as you increase the distance between yourself and the source.

LF radiation can be measured using an LF meter, often called a Gauss meter. You will observe that after moving half a meter to 1 meter away from indoor electrical wiring or 1 meter to 1.5 meters away from an ELF source such as a refrigerator ELF radiation levels will drop considerably. Please refer to subsequent sections for details on how to measure and protect yourself from ELF radiation. **NOTE:** The LF radiation exposure limit recommended by the 2012 Bioinitiative report is 1 Milligauss (mG) or 0.1 Micro-Tesla

Figure 2.1 Sources of Low Frequency (LF) Radiation

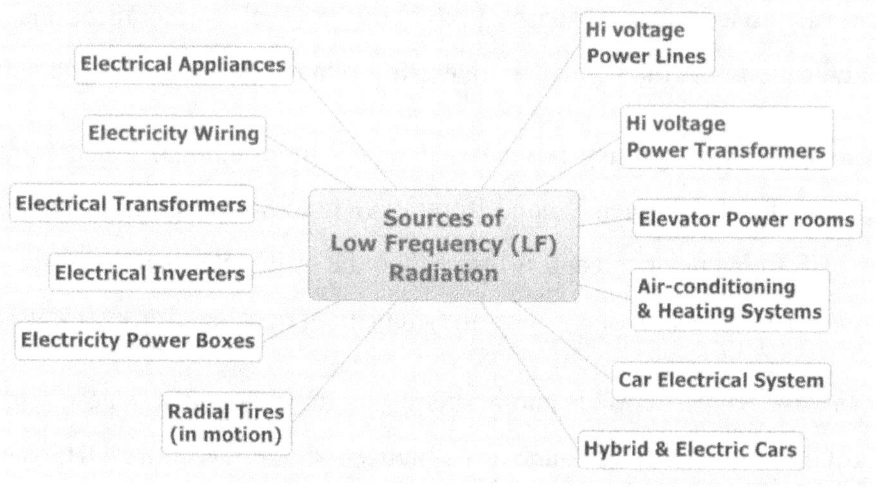

Radio Frequency (RF) Radiation

Unlike ELF radiation that is a by-product of electricity and electrical devices' normal operation, radio frequency (RF) radiation is generated and released intentionally into the environment. RF electromagnetic waves are used as carriers of information including data, audio and video. As such they serve a wide range of applications including radio stations, TV stations, cell-phone towers, DECT phones, cell phones, other mobile devices, Wi-Fi routers and Wi-Fi enabled devices, Bluetooth devices, smart meters, and radars.

Radio frequencies range from 3 KHz to 300 GHz - a very wide range of frequencies. However, we are mainly interested in those parts of the radio spectrum that are common sources of RF electromagnetic radiation. The most commonly used EMF bands of RF radiation that affect us in daily life are:

- **Very High frequency (VHF)** - electromagnetic frequencies from 30 MHz to 300 MHz that are mostly used for FM radio and TV broadcasts, aircraft and maritime communication

- **Ultra-High frequency (UHF)** - electromagnetic frequencies from 300 MHz to 3000 MHz (3 GHz) that are mostly used for some TV broadcasts, microwave communications, radio astronomy, cell phones, wireless LAN, Bluetooth, GPS, two-way radios and microwave ovens.

- **Super High frequency (SHF)** - electromagnetic frequencies from 3 GHz to 300 GHz that are mostly used for wireless LAN, microwave communications, radar systems, communications satellites, satellite **television broadcasting and radio astronomy.**

- **Extremely high frequency (EHF)** is the ITU (International Telecommunication Union) designation for the frequency band from 30 GHz to 300 GHz. It constitutes the higher part of the SHF frequency band and is also called the millimeter band because the waves in this band have a wavelength of 1 - 10 millimeters and are called millimetre waves.

- **"Microwave frequencies"** is another term you may encounter. These range from 300 MHz to 100 GHz. Microwave frequencies actually include the entire UHF band and the lower part of the SHF band. In daily life we are mostly concerned with protecting ourselves from

Microwave frequencies as these include cell-phones, DECT phones, Wi-Fi, cell-phone towers and other microwave communication towers.

As described in a previous section the frequency of an electromagnetic wave indicates how many times per second the wave oscillates. Since wave-length is in inverse proportion to the frequency - the higher the frequency the shorter the wavelength and vice versa. Therefore, microwave RF has short wavelengths and consequently is much easier to block and shield against than LF waves. RF can be blocked and shielded provided suitable shielding technology and materials are applied correctly. Of course, as with any type of EMR, avoidance is always the best solution. For example, if you live close to a microwave communication tower you may be able to significantly reduce radiation levels inside your home using a range of RF shielding paints, fabrics and transparent films. However, it may prove to be expensive and labor intensive. Furthermore, whenever you step outside your home, you will be immediately exposed to the radiation emitted by the microwave transmission tower. So living close to a powerful RF hazard ultimately increases your EMR exposure levels regardless of the protective measures you use.

NOTE: For RF radiation outdoor exposure the 2007 Bioinitiative Report recommended a limit of $0.1 \ \mu W/cm^2$. On the other hand, in the updated 2012 Bioinitiative Report a precautionary level of between 0.0003 µW/cm2 to 0.0006 µW/cm2 was recommended.

As you can see the 2012 Bioinitiative Report has taken a much more stringent approach than in the 2007 Bioinitiative Report. On the other hand, safety levels used by various regulatory bodies today are still based on the "Thermal Effect Threshold" established over 50 years ago. The thermal effect is based on electromagnetic radiation's ability to cause a rise in temperature of living tissue. However, the 2012 Bioinitiative Report cites numerous studies conducted over the past 15 years that have identified numerous morbid bio-effects well below the "Thermal Effect threshold". These findings raise serious doubts regarding existing safety standards.

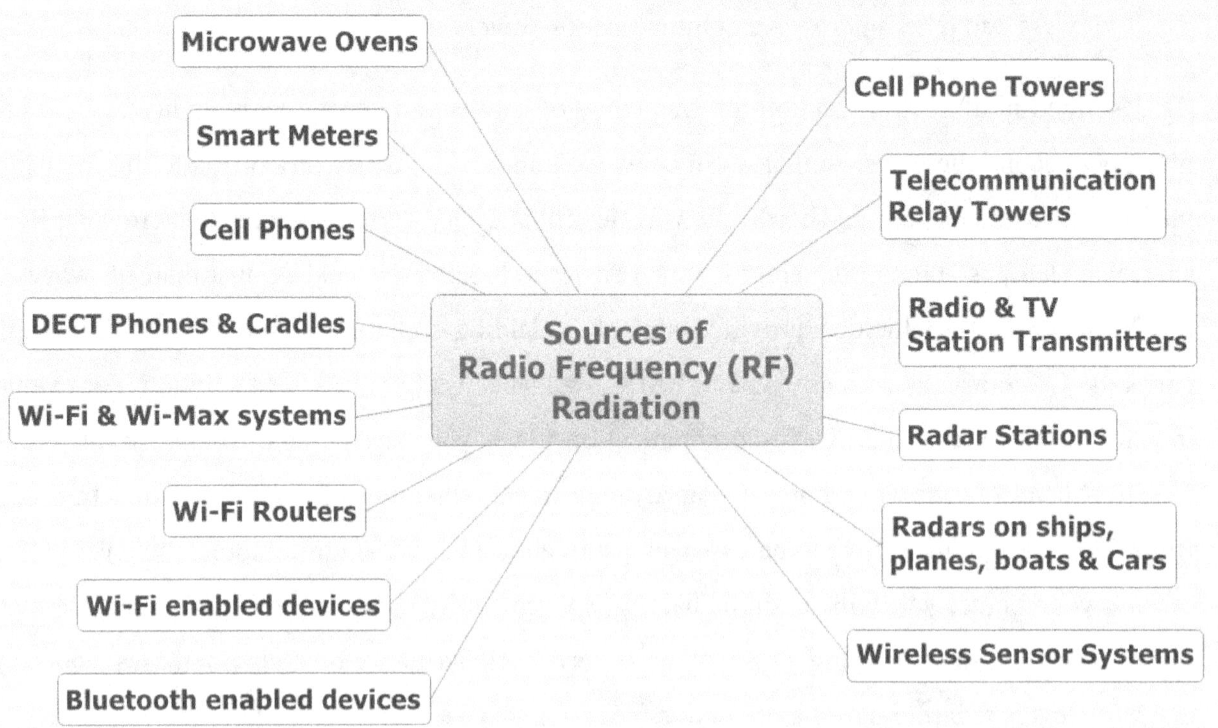

Figure 2.2 – Sources of RF radiatio

Image 2.1 - A Typical Cell Phone Tower

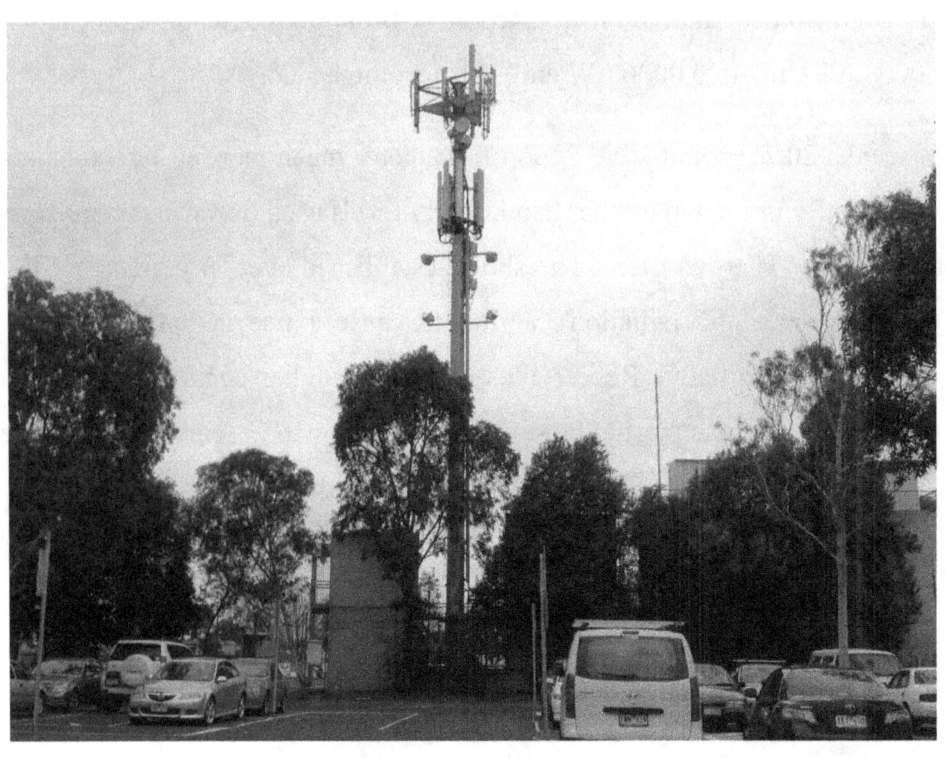

What is "Dirty Electricity" (DE)?

Dirty electricity is much less understood than LF or RF radiation despite the fact that several studies have linked dirty electricity to very serious health problems including cancer. Dirty electricity has been around for quite some time probably since the introduction of electricity. However, the introduction of electronic devices and wireless technology has contributed not only to an exponential increase in RF radiation levels but also to a significant increase in "Dirty Electricity" and the radiation it generates.

In its "normal" state the electricity supplied to our homes is a simple alternating current (**AC**). This current is generated by alternating voltage (**VAC**). The maximum voltage values in the homes depend on the country you live in (240 - 220 Volts or 110-100 Volts). The voltage in high voltage power transmission lines is much higher in order to reduce energy losses along the way. The AC has a frequency of 60 cycles per second (60 Hz) or 50 cycles per second (50 Hz) depending on the country you live in. Viewed on an oscilloscope, "clean" electricity looks like a nice sine wave. Dirty electricity is created when harmonics and transient micro-surges superimpose themselves (take a ride or piggyback) on top of the "clean" electrical current. These contaminating signals have much higher frequencies ranging from hundreds of Hz to hundreds of KHz. Viewed on an oscilloscope dirty electricity looks quite messy as the basic AC sine wave is covered with a lot of irregular spikes. These harmonics and micro-surges are like parasites attaching themselves to a dog's back and their effect on health can be just as bad if not worse.

How is "dirty electricity" created in the first place?

This is where things start getting complicated. There is no single source but rather a multitude of sources that contribute to the contamination of our electrical system and the creation of dirty electricity. Some of the contaminating sources are within the home or office and therefore within our control and some are external and enter our homes piggybacking on top of the AC supplied by the utility company.

Here are common sources of dirty electricity:

1. Significant amount of dirty electricity enters our homes via the main power supply. This is because the electricity grid outside has already been contaminated by various sources of high frequency signals. These signals may be generated by a range of electrical and electronic devices that are connected to the grid somewhere. They are like factories upstream that dump their toxic waste and pollute the river from which you get your drinking water downstream. The utility companies can significantly reduce the contamination by installing special low pass filters between the grid and the consumer. Perhaps consumer demand for such filters would encourage the utility companies to introduce these filters as standard equipment.

2. Electricity power cables also serve as antennas since they are made of highly conductive copper. They pick up radio frequency (**RF**) signals that happen to cross their path. For example: Radio, TV and microwave signals. Cell phone towers and other telecommunication towers that transmit microwave radiation are being erected everywhere. They are saturating the environment with EMF of varying frequencies. The electromagnetic waves are picked up by electrical power cables and electrical wiring. The electricity running through the cables becomes "dirty" as all sorts of signals superimpose themselves on the "clean" AC. Contaminated "dirty electricity" then enters our homes via the grid. In other words, even if you don't live right next to a cell phone tower, you may still be exposed to its harmful effects via the grid. In his book on dirty electricity Dr. Sam Milham gives an example of a public school in the US that had a telecommunication tower installed on its grounds. The level of dirty electricity in the classrooms was directly related to the distance to the tower. An association was found between cancer rates and the levels of dirty electricity in the classrooms.

3. Electronic devices generate high frequency electromagnetic pulses. Many of these devices do not have adequate filters to isolate them from the electrical network, so they pollute our electrical network with a range of high frequency pulses. These pulses superimpose on the clean electricity thus creating dirty electricity.

4. Some innocent looking electrical components are also responsible for contaminating our

electrical network with dirty electricity. For example: Dimmer switches, fluorescent lamps and even compact fluorescent lamps (**CFLs**). You may be doing the right thing for the environment, by using "green" energy saving CFLs but at the same time you may also be creating harmful "dirty electricity" in your home.

Figure 2.3 Sources of Dirty Electricity (DE)

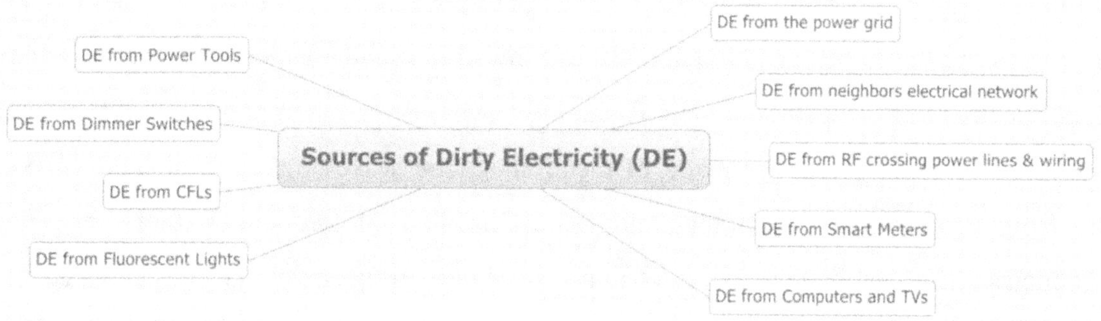

Why should I care about dirty electricity?

So what is the big deal about the "clean" electrical current becoming a little "dirty"? After all, electrical and electronic devices seem to be working OK. Well, here is the problem: Studies conducted by various scientists, most notably Dr. Sam Milham and Dr. Magda Havas have found a clear association (i.e. a connection or a link) between dirty electricity and a host of health disorders including cancer, autoimmune diseases and chronic fatigue. You can read about Dr. Milham's findings in his book Dirty electricity, and about Dr. Magda Havas' findings in her book Public Health SOS.

Actually dirty electricity itself is not the problem but rather the electromagnetic fields (EMF) that it generates. So-called "clean" electricity also generates an electromagnetic field with a frequency of 50 Hz or 60 Hz (depending on the frequency of the AC itself). This type of EMF is called extra low frequency (ELF). If you measure the ELF created around an electricity conducting wire, you will see that it is high only in close proximity to the wire, but the intensity drops off rapidly as you move further away. However, when it comes to dirty electricity the electrical wiring system of your house acts as an antenna transmitting EMF with much higher frequencies and these propagate throughout the entire home or building.

Technology and increasing levels of electromagnetic radiation

Technology keeps racing ahead. It provides many benefits but also exposes us to very serious health risks. One of the by-products of modern technology is the very inconvenient truth of air pollution and global warming. A less publicized but very serious problem is the fact that electricity and wireless technologies are creating a thick invisible cloud of electromagnetic radiation also called "Electrosmog". Electromagnetic Radiation (EMR) is the inherent energy of Electromagnetic Fields (EMF). These fields are made of electromagnetic waves traveling at light speed moving away from their source. Electromagnetic waves oscillate at frequencies that range from Low Frequencies (LF) generated by electricity to Radio frequencies (RF) generated by radio transmitters, microwave telecommunication and radar stations at the higher end of the scale. Just like the waves in the ocean electromagnetic waves also carry substantial amounts of energy. This energy is called Electromagnetic Energy. Unlike ocean waves, electromagnetic waves are invisible to the naked eye and cannot be felt or sensed by most people despite the fact that they have the ability to penetrate every cell of our bodies.

The link between the Internet and EMF

Internet traffic is increasing rapidly. More and more of this traffic is received and transmitted by mobile devices including smart phones, tablets, laptops and similar devices. To support an exponentially growing stream of data the telecommunication companies are rolling out more and more cell phone towers and various types of antennas are popping up on roof tops and even within large buildings (often very cleverly concealed). The coverage of **Wi-Fi** and **Wi-Max** networks is also being extended continuously. All of this is resulting in a substantial increase in ambient electromagnetic radiation creating a dense cloud of Electrosmog everywhere. Unlike a real cloud, the Electrosmog is not only outside us. It also penetrates our bodies 24/7 whether we like it or not. We are literally transparent to electromagnetic radiation as it goes straight through us just like light goes through a clear glass window penetrating every corner.

Factors affecting EMR exposure

The amount of radiation that reaches us and enters our body depends on various factors including the following:

1. The power of the transmitting source

2. The frequency/wavelength of the source

3. The shape and size of the transmitting source

4. The distance from the transmitting source

5. Barriers between the source and our body that may deflect, absorb or redirect the electromagnetic field

6. The grounding situation in our living/work space

7. The grounding situation of our own body

8. Personal physiological make-up

Effects of Non-Ionizing Electromagnetic Radiation

The 2012 Bioinitiative Report is a very comprehensive report that covers the science, public health, public policy and global response to the growing health issue of chronic exposure to electromagnetic fields (and radio frequency radiation (**RFR**). It is an update to a similar report prepared in 2007. It has been prepared by 29 independent scientists and health experts from many countries. The 2012 Update covers around 1800 new studies on bio-effects and adverse health effects of electromagnetic fields (power lines, electrical wiring, appliances etc.) and wireless technologies (cell and cordless phones, cell towers, Wi-Fi, wireless laptops, wireless routers, baby monitors, surveillance systems, 'smart meters' etc.) Both LF and RF electromagnetic radiation (EMR) were thought to be mostly benign, as they are non-ionizing (i.e. do not knock out electrons out of atoms) but a growing body of scientific evidence supports the disturbing conclusions of the 2012 Bioinitiative report - briefly summarized below:

Existing safety standards – are they adequate?

Every country has its own EMF safety standards and they vary considerably. The Bioinitiative report recommends reassessing existing safety standards for radiation from wireless devices. The scientists that wrote the report believe that most existing safety standards are not only inadequate but also fundamentally flawed. This is because they are based on very outdated research conducted in the 1950s to establish safety standards for non-ionizing electromagnetic radiation. Non-ionizing electromagnetic radiation is so called because it is not able to knock out electrons from their orbits around the nuclei of atoms. In other words, it cannot cause an atom to become an ion (i.e. - an electrically charged particle). In the early days researchers thought that if electromagnetic radiation does not ionize atoms then it can be considered safe as long as it does not result in a significant rise in the temperature of living tissues, a phenomenon called the "Thermal Effect" upon which microwave ovens are based. This line of outdated thinking still determines existing electromagnetic radiation safety standards. Other possible effects are not taken into consideration. However, the 2012 Bioinitiative report cites 1800 studies reporting a wide range of morbid bio-effects caused by Electromagnetic Radiation (EMR) well below the thermal effect threshold. The Bioinitiative report maintains that permissible radiation levels in most countries are already 1000 to 10000 times too high. In a 2011 World Health Organization (WHO) International Agency for Research on Cancer (IARC) press release, all radio frequency electromagnetic fields were classified *as a possible carcinogen to humans*[3]. In 2011 The Parliamentary Assembly Council of Europe released a resolution on the potential dangers of electromagnetic fields and their effect on the environment. The resolution states that: *'Telecommunications and mobile telephony, appear to have more or less potentially harmful, non-thermal, biological effects on plants, insects and animals as well as the human body, even when exposed to levels that are below the official threshold values.*[1]*'*

It may take some time for the full consequences of EMF exposure to become recognized by the scientific community and government. Unfortunately, by that time many may develop serious health conditions with implications on private and public health. Furthermore, a growing number of people called 'Electro Hypersensitive' (EHS) are already presenting to their doctors with various complaints related to the adverse effects EMFs and the numbers of EHS are rising rapidly. Therefore, the time to deal with the problem is NOW.

Image 2.2 – A combination of LF and RF pollution

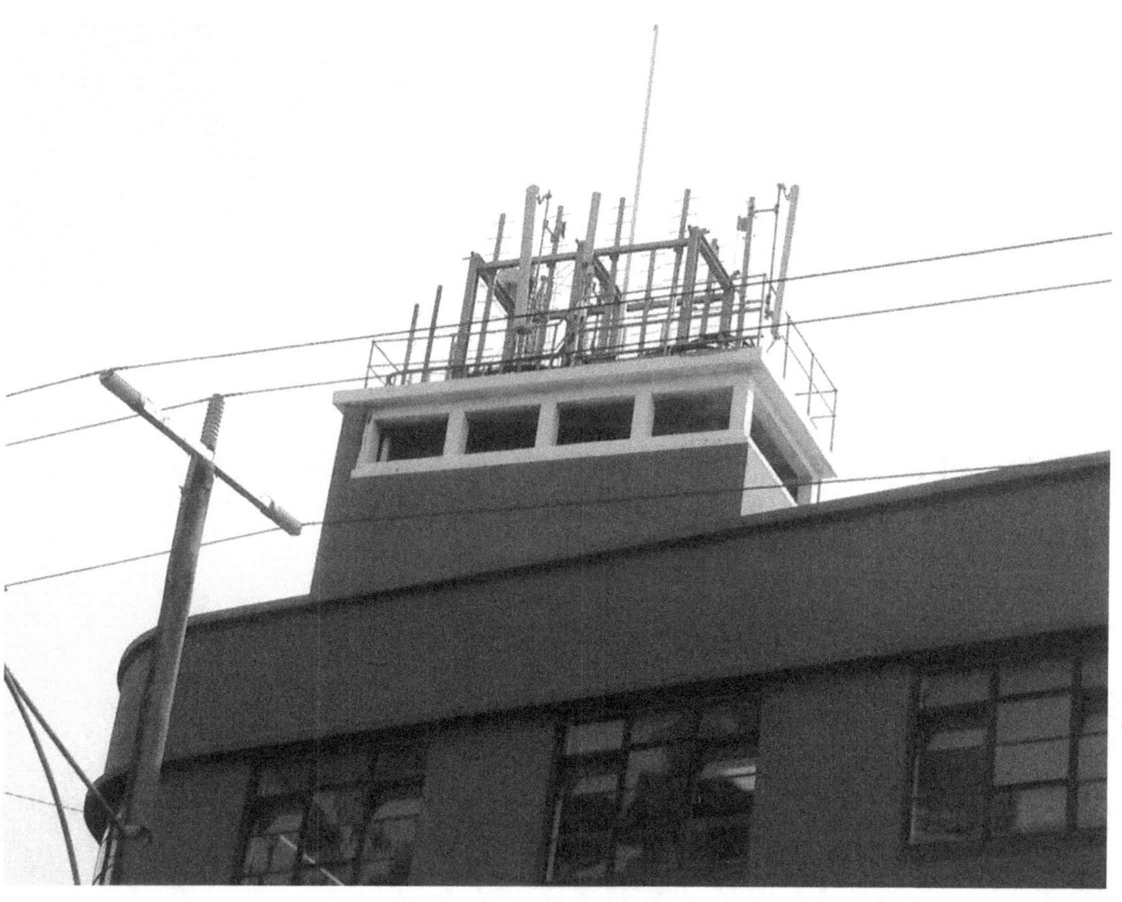

3. 5G AND THE 'INTERNET OF THINGS' (IOT)

We'll address the following:

- What is 5G?

- Is 5G very different from 3G and 4G?

- 5G frequency bands

- 5G antennas and technologies

- How will 5G interact with other emerging technologies?

- Will 5G result in higher radiation (EMR) levels?

- How will 5G impact health?

- How will 5G impact privacy and security?

- How will 5G impact human rights?

- 5G protection - in chapter 26

What is 5G?

5G is the fifth generation standard for broadband cellular networks, originally intended to supersede the existing 4G standard although in reality will not replace 4G in the coming years but rather, will be superimposed on existing 4G networks and also be used in new applications such as the 'Internet of Things'. 5G roll-out started in 2019 and it has been accelerating rapidly. 5G frequencies will be transmitted from cellular antennas, satellites, Wi-Fi routers and mobile phones.

Is 5G different from 3G and 4G?

In short – yes and no! Like 3G and 4G, 5G is a cellular network technology that divides service areas into geographical sections called cells. 5G allows increased bandwidth and higher data throughput especially in the millimeter wave bands. This translates to much faster download and upload speeds, reduced connection delays and lag time, a much larger number of mobile devices that can be serviced per geographical cell.

5G frequency bands

5G frequency bands can be divided into low, middle and high frequency bands. Existing 4G frequency bands have wavelengths that are several centimeters long. The low and middle 5G bands are similar to existing 4G frequency bands. At present:

- **600-850 MHz** has been allocated to the **low 5G frequency band**

- **2.5 - 3.7 GHz** has been allocated to the **middle 5G frequency band**

- **25-39 GHz** has been allocated to the **high 5G frequency band.** The high frequency 5G frequency waves are several millimeters long (and hence called millimeter waves).

- Higher 5G frequency millimeter wave bands may be added in the future.

5G Applications

5G will be used by cell phone networks, using new cellphones and cellphone towers and new Wi-Fi routers. It will also be used for a wide range of new applications and services. Major internet service providers intend to offer 5G connectivity in addition to and in some cases instead of fiber optic cable or copper wire ADSL connectivity. Switching from fiber optic and copper cables to 5G radio frequencies will make life easier for service providers and increase their profit margins. Just think of all the cables they will not have to install and connect to every house and apartment.

The 'Internet of Things' (IoT)

IoT Stands for a network of devices, appliances and sensors linked via Wi-Fi networks and the internet. These may include sensors, security and surveillance systems, air-conditioning systems, audiovisual systems, appliances (e.g. refrigerators, stoves, washing machines)and even disposable consumer goods and will be an important part of 'smart homes', 'smart buildings', 'smart cities', 'smart healthcare', 'smart traffic control', 'smart manufacturing and industrial systems' etc. All these will be communicating and exchanging information constantly using 5G technologies and causing a dramatic increase in the level of EMR both indoors and outdoors. IoT will operate via 5G Wi-Fi and mobile networks inside and outside buildings, homes, offices, hospitals, factories, public and private transport, government and city services etc.

5G from Satellites

Tens of thousands of mini-satellites are being launched into orbits around Earth to provide high frequency 5G connectivity around the globe. In other words EMR will rain on us from the sky as well.

5G and increasing radiation levels

5G will dramatically increase available bandwidth and hence data throughput as well as number of serviceable devices per cellular geographical area. It will also utilise a much wider range of radio frequencies. Because higher frequencies (millimeter waves) have a shorter service range, many more antennas are needed. In densely populated urban areas "small cell" base station 5G antennas may be installed on or next to every second or third building, utility poles, lamp posts etc. High band 5G are more prone to obstruction by solid objects (e.g. walls, trees), moisture, rain etc. To overcome this, transmitted radiation levels have to be increased dramatically. A technology called Massive MIMO (Multiple input Multiple output) has been introduced in 4G in conjunction with a technology called 'Beam-forming'. These technologies will also be used in 5G millimeter wave bands. MIMO uses multiple antennas in each cell antenna array and 'Beam-forming' calculates the best route and antenna combination to concentrate the energy targeted at a specific device in order maximize performance and overcome the difficulty 5G millimeter wave bands have in penetrating solid objects (e.g. walls, trees, cars etc.). The resulting 5G beam is very concentrated and has higher EMR levels. It is transmitted intermittently on demand basis as opposed to the 4G EMR that is transmitted continuously from base station antennas. The 4G and 5G EMR will overlap as new small cell antenna arrays utilize both. Expect rapid wide-scale implementation of 5G and related technologies, such as the Internet of Things (IoT), Satellite EMF raining from the sky, 5G and 4G antenna arrays showering us with EMR on every street corner, 5G routers and mobile devices inside homes, schools, offices, hospitals. This will result in a massive increase in EMR levels that is hard to predict accurately but expected to be thousands of times higher than existing levels, that are already much too high.

How will 5G impact health?

Insufficient research has been done on the bio-effects of 3G and 4G (centimeter wavelengths), mostly using animal models. As of early 2021, <u>no studies</u> have been published on the bio-effects of commercial 5G millimeter waves on humans, animals and plants. However, research has been conducted by governments, using millimeter waves, for developing various types of non-lethal weapons and significant bioeffects have been shown. With the launching of tens of thousands of 5G related satellites, there will literally be nowhere left to hide and humans, animals, plants and the environment, will be affected not only in urban areas but everywhere around the planet. There is no way to even try to predict the magnitude of the impending 5G EMR catastrophe. In humans this may result in various health disorders. In the animal and plant kingdoms it will superimpose on global warming and pollution to accelerate environmental damage, loss of biodiversity and dysregulation of the food chains. Wild pollinators including bees, birds, bats and others, affect 87 percent of the leading crops around the world. These pollinators include 20,000 types of bees. Massive loss of bee colonies, declining numbers and productivity has been reported around the globe. This has been attributed to pesticides, parasites and weather changes but some scientific studies have shown that cell phone EMR resulted in declining colony numbers and honey production. All these may result in decline in food production around the globe.

How will 5G impact privacy and security?

The 5G standard was designed with improved security in mind compared to 4G. However, it also has vulnerabilities that are being discovered with time. 5G allows pinpointing the location of a cell phone in real time with great accuracy. This of course has advantages but also disadvantages if the phone is hacked. However, the greatest threats to privacy and security come from the Internet of Things (IoT). The rapid rollout of 5G and IoT will trigger the development and production of billions of devices, gadgets and sensors and most of them insecure and easy to hack. This will put your privacy and data at great risk. Hackers, organizations and governments will be able to monitor your every move and conversations in real time, collect information on your lifestyle, habits, use of appliances, resources, and just about anything that can be picked up by sensors and transmitted via the internet.

How will 5G impact human rights?

We will be facing the same human right issues with 5G as with 4G but on a much larger scale. So far there has been limited success in preventing cell phone towers installation in urban areas, but at least being located several hundred meters apart allows people to live as far away as they can. 5G antennas will be much closer and greater in numbers. So far the telecom industry has the upper hand and courts are usually turning down objections and appeals by councils and individuals. The rollout of 5G antennas everywhere compared to 3G and 4G much lower antenna density is presented to the courts as more 'democratic' and equitable where everyone is exposed to EMR in the same way.

How to protect yourself from 5G

Some aspects of 5G protection are similar to 4G cell phone and Wi-Fi protection and some are unique to 5G and will be discussed in chapter 26.

4. EMF PROTECTION BASICS

There are several EMF protection principles that you can implement immediately to protect yourself from EMF hazards. After reading this section you will be ready to dive into each of the components of your EMF protection action plan in detail.There are several methods to deal with EMF/EMR and in most cases for achieving the best results we need to combine several methods because often no method is totally effective on its own. Different types of EMF/EMR hazards (listed above) also require different protection solutions. Understanding the basic concepts described in this section will help you design and implement an effective EMF self defense plan.

When electromagnetic waves propagate through outer space and do not come into contact with an object, they continue to spread undiminished. However, on planet Earth any type of EMF is bound to come into contact with object(s). These include the earth and its topographical features, any life form that grows or lives on the surface of the earth and of course men made structures and equipment. Any of these objects may absorb, reflect or redirect EMF. Most objects usually absorb some of the radiation, reflect some of it and allow the remaining radiation to go through and continue to travel on the other side of the obstacle. Some objects behave as a transparent film; in other words, they allow most of the radiation to go straight through them just like light shining through a window.

EMFs with different frequencies also interact differently with a range of materials and fabrics. For example, a metallic mesh may reflect a significant percentage of microwave RF radiation but at the same time is totally ineffective at blocking LF (low frequency) radiation.

Choosing EMF Protection Methods

Our choice of EMF protection methods depends on the following factors:

- Type of EMF (i.e. LF, RF or caused by dirty electricity)

- Level of EMF exposure (i.e. low, mid-range or high levels)

- Frequency of EMF exposure (i.e. rare, occasional or constant)

- Type of object or environment we are trying to protect (i.e. home, back yard, office, car, adult, child, baby, pet, equipment etc.)

Main EMF Protection Methods

These are the main strategies for dealing with EMF/EMR:

1. Avoidance

2. Reduction

3. Reflection

4. Absorption

5. Redirection

6. Suppression

7. Cancellation

Figure 4.1 Basic EMF Protection Strategies

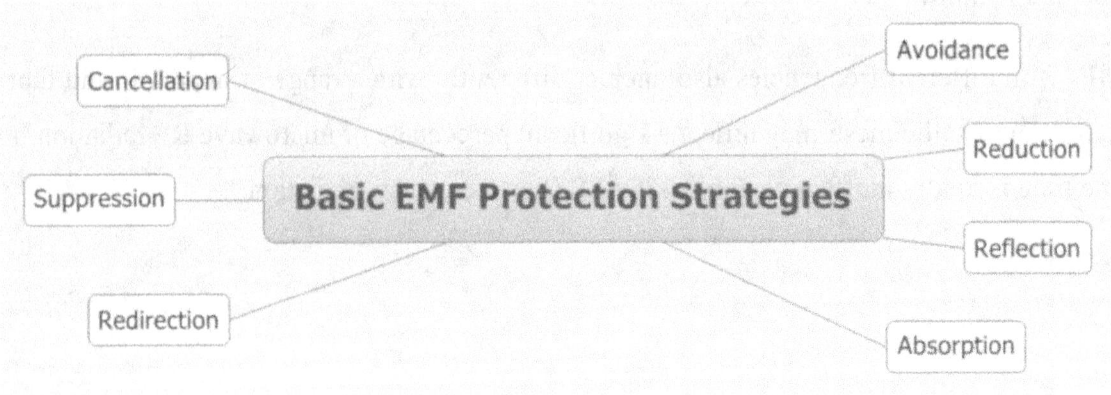

Let us look at each of these methods in more detail in order to get a better understanding of how each fits into the overall EMF protection strategy.

Avoidance

Avoidance simply means to avoid creating EMF fields around you and to avoid being where EMF fields are present. Avoidance is the most obvious and effective method of dealing with EMF/EMR. However, it is often very difficult to completely avoid EMF unless you choose to live your life very far from modern civilization without using any kind of electrical or electronic devices. Having said that you can still apply a range of measures that will help you avoid much of the EMF/EMR you are currently exposed to. These steps are discussed in detail in subsequent sections. For now, let's just give ten examples of EMF avoidance:

1. Avoid living or working next to high voltage power lines.
2. Avoid living or working next to cell phone towers.
3. Avoid sleeping or working close to power boxes and powerful electrical appliances (e.g. refrigerators)
4. Avoid sleeping or working near electrical wiring.
5. Only use cell-phones in emergencies
6. Avoid using Wi-Fi at home. Use wired Ethernet connections instead.
7. Avoid using Wi-Fi enabled devices.
8. Avoid going for a walk under power lines
9. Avoid going for a walk close to cell-phone towers
10. Avoid frequent commuting on crowded trains or buses.

From the examples we have just given it becomes obvious that EMF avoidance may require making changes in daily habits, life style, living location and even occupation. Depending on your circumstances some of these measures may be easy to implement and some may require making considerable sacrifices. Some may not be possible to implement at all. And this is exactly the reason why we also need to use other EMF protection measures. They are all there for situations where avoidance is simply impractical or impossible.

Reduction

Reduction simply means - that if you cannot completely avoid EMR exposure then at least try to reduce it. Reduction is therefore a type of damage control strategy. Here are ten examples of how reduction is applied in real life:

1. Reduce your cell-phone air-time by using your phone less frequently and keeping the calls short.

2. Reduce EMR exposure by keeping the cell phone as far away from your body when making a call. You can increase your distance by using a speaker-phone or an air tube headset. Other sections discuss why this may dramatically reduce your EMR exposure.

3. Keep your cell phone away from your body when not using it. For example, put it in your purse instead of carrying it on your belt or in your pocket.

4. Reduce Wi-Fi usage by using it less frequently and only when there are no other alternatives (as discussed in other sections) and even then keep it short. For example: Connect to the network, download your email quickly and disconnect.

5. Reduce EMR exposure by sitting or standing as far as possible from any source of ELF EMF/EMR (e.g. electrical cables, power-boxes, refrigerators, computers, electric clocks and other devices).

6. Reduce EMR exposure by sitting or standing as far as possible from any source of RF EMF/EMR (e.g. cell-phone antennas, Wi-Fi routers, cell phones, Wi-Fi enabled devices etc.)

7. When located close to a cell phone tower, stay indoors and do not venture outside.

8. Do not drive on roads that have hi voltage power lines running alongside.

9. When going for a walk around the block do not walk under power cables. Cross the street and proceed along the opposite side of the street.

10. If you are living in a house or apartment that is close to power lines, try to relocate your sleeping and living space to rooms most distant from the power lines.

Reflection

Reflection means to bounce EMF/EMR away from a person or an object. This method is only effective for RF type EMF/EMR. This method will not work for LF type EMF because of its very long wavelength.

In the real world every material or object reflects some EMF, absorbs some EMF and lets the rest go through. You can get a better understanding of how this works by comparing it to what happens with sunlight. Sunlight warms us because our body absorbs part of the sun's electromagnetic spectrum resulting in a heating effect. We can see objects because sunlight is reflected back from these objects and an image is formed on our retina. Different objects appear to have different colors because they reflect different parts of the visible light spectrum. The reflected part of the spectrum is the color we see (e.g. blue). EMF reflective materials are so called because they reflect most of the EMF/EMR that hits them. EMF reflective materials typically have a zone of the RF spectrum for which they are very effective reflectors and the efficacy declines as the frequency goes outside that zone. EMF reflective materials may also absorb part of the EMR and allow the rest to go through. All these parameters have to be taken into consideration when selecting the appropriate reflecting material to resolve your EMF/EMR problem. There is a wide range of EMF reflective materials that can be used including:

1. RF shielding paints used mainly to paint internal and external walls and also partitions.

2. RF shielding fabrics used mainly to make curtains for windows and doors, canopies for bedtime protection, clothing for personal EMF protection, cases for shielding cell-phones and pads for shielding laptops and tablets.

3. RF shielding transparent films for shielding glass windows or doors.

Note: LF cannot be reflected effectively due to its long wavelength and is much harder to deal with as described below.

Absorption

All materials absorb part of the EMR that reaches them. Unfortunately, the human body absorbs a significant proportion of the EMR and this results in various undesirable bio-effects. EMR absorptive materials absorb a significant percentage of the EMR that reaches them. The energy is then dissipated to the environment as heat. There is a wide range of EMF absorbing materials that can be used including:

1. RF paints are used mainly to coat internal and external walls and also partitions are used mainly for reflection but also absorb part of the EMR.

2. RF absorbing wallpaper used mainly to cover walls and partitions

Redirection

This method is used mainly in special cell-phone cases that are designed to redirect a significant percent of the radiation emitted by the phone's internal antenna away from the user via an external antenna built into the back of the special case. This results in a reduction of EMR exposure and also an improvement in the phone's reception and transmission.

Suppression

The EMF created by dirty electricity is very hard to block. However, the good news is that dirty electricity can be suppressed easily by installing dirty electricity filters. These filters clean the electricity by filtering out micro-surges and high frequency transients and redirecting that energy to the ground.

Cancellation

Some very expensive active systems have been designed to cancel specific LF fields by generating a field with the same frequency and opposite polarity. These devices will cancel the field only in a limited area for which the cancellation effect was calibrated. Anywhere outside that zone you would actually be exposed to higher EMF. This solution is not applicable for most common situations and applications.

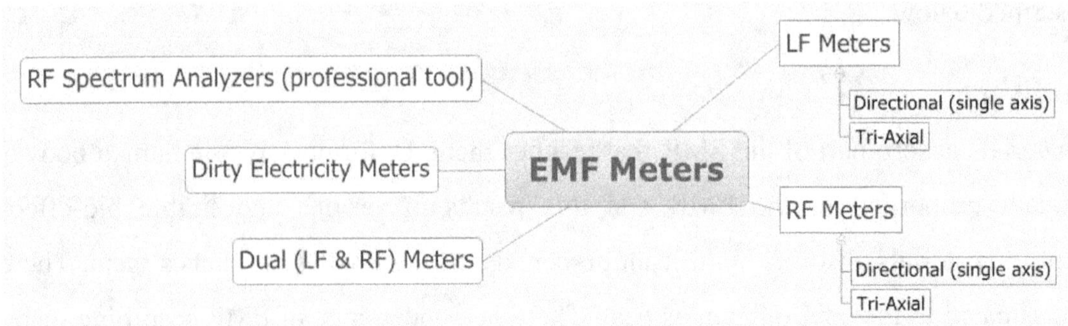

Figure 4.2 EMF meters

5 LOW FREQUENCY (LF) EMR PROTECTION

LF/ELF electromagnetic fields are everywhere

In every home or office there you can always find several sources of LF/ELF including:

1. Electric power box(s)

2. Electrical wiring

3. Electrical appliances such as air conditioning systems, refrigerators, ovens, vacuum cleaners, heaters etc.

4. In apartment buildings there may also be sources outside the apartments such as central air conditioning systems, central heating systems, elevator power rooms etc.

LF upper safety limit - Quoting from the conclusions of the 2012 Bioinitiative report:

'As one step in the direction of precaution, measures should be implemented to guarantee that exposure due to transmission and distribution lines are below an average of about 1 mG. This value is arbitrary at present and only supported by the fact that in many studies this level has been chosen as a reference.'

Basic LF protection strategies

Dealing with LF radiation can be quite difficult especially if radiation levels are high (above 2 Milligauss). LF fields are strong at the source but dissipate rapidly as you move away. Therefore, a combination of the avoidance and reduction methods should be attempted first. For example:

1. If there is a power box on the other side of the wall move your bed as far away from that wall as possible. Perhaps even to a different room.

2. Don't spend much time sitting next to the refrigerator, heater, fan etc.

3. If the building's central air-conditioning system or elevator power room is located directly next to, above or below your apartment and EMR readings are high you may consider relocation.

4. However, when avoidance and reduction are not possible, you may need to use special protection materials. These are usually in the form of plates and flexible sheets and foils made of special metal alloys. These materials are very expensive. Some of these materials are composed of several layers each having different and complementary deflection, blocking and absorbing properties. Blocking significant LF radiation (above 2 Milligauss) should be done by LF protection professionals. LF radiation protection is a specialty within EMF protection. Many EMF consultants have more experience with RF radiation protection and less experience with LF radiation protection so you need to find the right person for the job.

Measuring low frequency EMF - What are we actually measuring?

Measuring ELF radiation is the first step you need to take before planning and implementing your EMF protection strategy. Measuring ELF is relatively easy but needs to be done methodically to ensure accuracy. This section will take you through the steps you need to follow in order to get a good picture of ELF radiation in your home or office.

LF spans the range of 3Hz to 30 KHz. LF is further divided as follows:

- Extremely low frequency (ELF) - are electromagnetic frequencies from 3 Hz to 3Kz.

- Very low frequency (VLF) - are electromagnetic frequencies from 3 KHz to 30 KHz

- The frequency of alternating current (AC) is 50 Hz or 60 Hz depending on the country you live in. The EMF generated by AC oscillate at 50 Hz or 60 Hz respectively. So naturally we are mostly interested in this sub-band of ELF as defined above.

Getting the right LF meter

There are a variety of LF meters (sometimes called Gauss meters) on the market. For DIY there is no need to get a professional level meter as it can be quite expensive. On the other hand, I don't recommend getting a cheap meter as most are of poor quality and may not perform reliably. There are plenty of good meters in the mid-price range. I do not recommend using a "Ghost detector" for this purpose.

Here are the functions you should look for when buying an EMF meter:

1. There are basically two types of meters: **Single-axis (directional) meters and tri-axial meters**. Directional meters only measure the EMR level along one axis (for example the X axis) whereas the tri-axial meters measure radiation levels along each of the three axes (X, Y and Z) in relation to the meter's orientation at the time of taking a reading. Tri-axial meters also have a built in algorithm that sums up the results from all three axes to approximate the real radiation level. Tri-axial meters have an advantage over directional meters. They save time and are more convenient to use. With single-axis directional meters you need to tilt the meter slowly in different directions until you get the maximum reading. This may be time consuming and may decrease accuracy.

2. Some meters can measure both components of the electromagnetic field, namely – the **electric and the magnetic components** while most LF meters only measure the magnetic component. These are often called Gauss meters. You will be able to tell what kind of meter it is by looking at the units on the scales. Magnetic fields are expressed by Gauss, Milligauss (mG), Tesla or Micro-Tesla. Electric fields are usually expressed in volts per meter (V/m). For most applications measuring the magnetic component will provide enough information.

3. The two common units used to measure LF magnetic fields are the **Milligauss and the micro-Tesla.** One micro-Tesla equals 10 Milligauss therefore the conversion is easy - you simply need to multiply the reading in microTesla by 10 to get the equivalent in Milligauss. However, in scientific reports and literature the Milligauss is used more

often. Therefore, ideally your meter would provide a reading in Milligauss or in both units. Often there is a button that allows selecting between these units.

4. Another useful feature is the **MAX/MIN** function. This function allows determining minimum and maximum radiation levels within a specified time frame. It is especially important to be able to determine maximum value if the field intensity fluctuates (e.g. in refrigerators and other systems operated by thermostats).

5. Another useful function is the **HOLD** function that freezes the value on the display and enables you to write it down.

6. Another useful function is the **REC** function that enables you to store results in the meter's memory and retrieve them later.

7. An important function is an **auto shut-down.** This function can be set to shut down the meter if it is inactive for a pre-set length of time. This will significantly extend the life of the battery.

Making a diagram of your house, apartment or office

After getting the right meter, make a sketch of your apartment or house. A simple sketch will do. The sketch will help you record your readings and identify hotspots. The sketch needs to include the following elements:

1. Rooms

2. Location of hi voltage power cables and transformers outside your house

3. Location of the main power box

4. Location of the entry point of power lines coming from the street into the house

5. Electrical appliances in each room (refrigerator, oven, mini air-conditioning systems, heating systems, lights with dimmer switches, computer equipment etc.)

6. Power sockets in each room

7.   Extension power cords and power boards running from power sockets.

8.   Locations where neighbors may have LF radiation emitting devices on the other side of a wall (e.g. power boxes, refrigerators, electric heaters etc.)

Radiation measurements in each of the rooms

Levels of ELF radiation may vary considerably within a single room. Therefore, you need to take several measurements in each room. As a minimum I suggest that you perform the following measurements:

1.   Measure radiation levels next to the main power box and on the other side of the wall to which the power-box is attached.

2.   Measure radiation levels next to the central air-conditioning unit (if you have one) outside the house and inside the house on the other side of the wall to which the system is attached.

3.   Measure radiation levels next to the solar system inverter unit (if you have one) outside the house and inside the house on the other side of the wall to which the inverter is attached. The measurement should be performed during the day-time, as at night the inverter may not be in operation. Solar system inverters often produce very substantial electromagnetic radiation of up to a 1000 Milligauss (about a thousand times higher than the upper safety limit).

4.   Measure radiation levels next to each of the electrical appliances.

5.   Measure radiation levels close to each dimmer switch when the light is on

6.   Measure radiation levels close to each power transformer leading to an electrical device when the device is ON. For example: transformers connected to laptops, printers, audio systems, TV screens .

7.   Measure radiation levels close to each power socket.

8.   Measure radiation levels close to each of the power boards when the extension cord is connected and the switch is ON.

9. Measure radiation levels in each of the beds where people normally sleep.

10. Measure radiation levels in the children's play areas.

11. Measure radiation levels in each of the armchairs and sofas where you spend time relaxing.

12. Measure radiation levels around your work desk.

13. Measure radiation levels at each of the four corners of each room, next to the wall halfway between the two corners and at the center of each room.

Using measurement results for identifying LF hazards

1. If significant portions of your house or office are saturated by high levels of LF/ELF this is not a good sign. The radiation may be coming from high tension power lines outside, a central air-conditioning system or an elevator power room close by. Protecting against such ELF hazards may be very expensive or even impossible. In such cases you may need to consider relocation. **REMEMBER:** Health is Wealth.

2. If you only detect ELF hotspots, in other words you do not detect an overall high level of ELF in your house or office then this means that you can probably work around the hotspots and protect yourself effectively against ELF.

3. Radiation level should not exceed 1 Milligauss. Ideally it should be below 0.5 Milligauss and below 0.25 Milligauss is even better. First - identify radiation hot spots. These are areas where the radiation is higher than 1 Milligauss. Try to determine the source. Is it an external source (e.g. power lines outside) or an internal source? Is the source concentrated in a small area (e.g. a power box) or a large area (e.g. an electric heating system with elements built in under the floor)?

4. How far away from the power-box, solar system inverter, air-conditioning system, and heating systems - do you have to move back until you measure safe radiation levels? What about the other side of the wall to which these units are attached?

5. Are there any hotspots in areas where people spend much time? For example, are there hot spots close to beds, desks, playrooms? Can beds, desks, armchairs, sofas, play areas

be rearranged so they are far from hotspots and within safe radiation level zones?

6. Is there any radiation emitting device that can be disconnected from the power supply most of the time (e.g. electric ovens and microwave ovens)?

7. Are fridges, freezers, air-conditioners, electric heaters emitting high levels of radiation? How far do you need to move back until your measurements show acceptable radiation levels? What about the other side of the wall? Do you need to reposition beds, armchairs, desks, tables located on the other side of the wall?

8. Are any of the transformers emitting high radiation levels? Are they emitting significantly higher levels than other transformers? How far from the transformer does radiation level become safe? Can the transformers be positioned further away from desks, tables, chairs, beds so people are not sitting close to them?

9. Can you detect hot spots next to any of the sockets, power boards, switches, dimmer switches?

Basic ELF reduction measures

After rearranging your sleep, work and living spaces in such a way that you and your family spend most of the time away from ELF hotspots and in safe low ELF zones you can take additional simple steps that may further reduce ELF radiation levels throughout your house:

1. Install a central demand switch next to your power-box. This switch automatically disconnects branches of your electrical network if they are not consuming electrical power. This prevents ELF from being generated throughout those parts of the electrical network and is especially useful at night.
   Note: The demand switch must be installed by a qualified electrician.

2. Replace old electrical sockets with sockets that have an on/off switch. Turn sockets OFF when the electrical device(s) plugged into that socket are not being used. This will reduce residual ELF from being generated by devices that are not being used and also extend their life.
   Note: The demand switch must be installed by a qualified electrician.

3. A simpler alternative to replacing sockets is getting electrical power-boards with safety switches. Turn the safety switches OFF when the electrical device(s) plugged into the power-board are not being used. Some power-boards have only one switch and others have a safety switch for each individual socket. These allow switching off devices that are not being used while still using others.

ELF/LF shielding

You may further reduce ELF levels using ELF shielding. Shielding should be the last resort as it can be expensive. Some forms of ELF shielding described below are best done when constructing or renovating houses as most electrical wiring is installed behind walls and above ceilings. Following are several LF shielding options. Minor LF electromagnetic sources ELF fields produced around electrical wiring and electrical appliances can often be shielded effectively. Shielding may not eliminate the EMR completely but may be able to lower it below the 1 mG upper safety limit as recommended by the 2012 Bioinitiative report.

1. Some paints can shield against low level ELF. These are suitable for relatively weak fields emanating from electrical wiring running through the walls. These paints are not suitable for stronger fields such as those produced by electric power boxes or electrical power cables outside the house.

2. Special LF blocking protective tubing and conduits are used for containing ELF radiation from electrical wiring. The wiring has to be inserted into these conduits. This work should be done by a certified experienced electrician only.

3. Special electrical wires are designed to maximize EMF cancellation and suppression using special internal configuration. These wires emit up to 90% less EMF than regular electric wires.

CAUTION:

1. You should not attempt to do any electrical work by yourself as this can be dangerous, may lead to electrocution or even death. This work should be done by a certified electrician only.

2. Shielding paints may require grounding. Grounding should only be installed by a certified electrician following manufacturer's instructions.

3. All electrical wiring should only be installed by a certified electrician

Figure 5.1 LF Radiation Protection Strategy

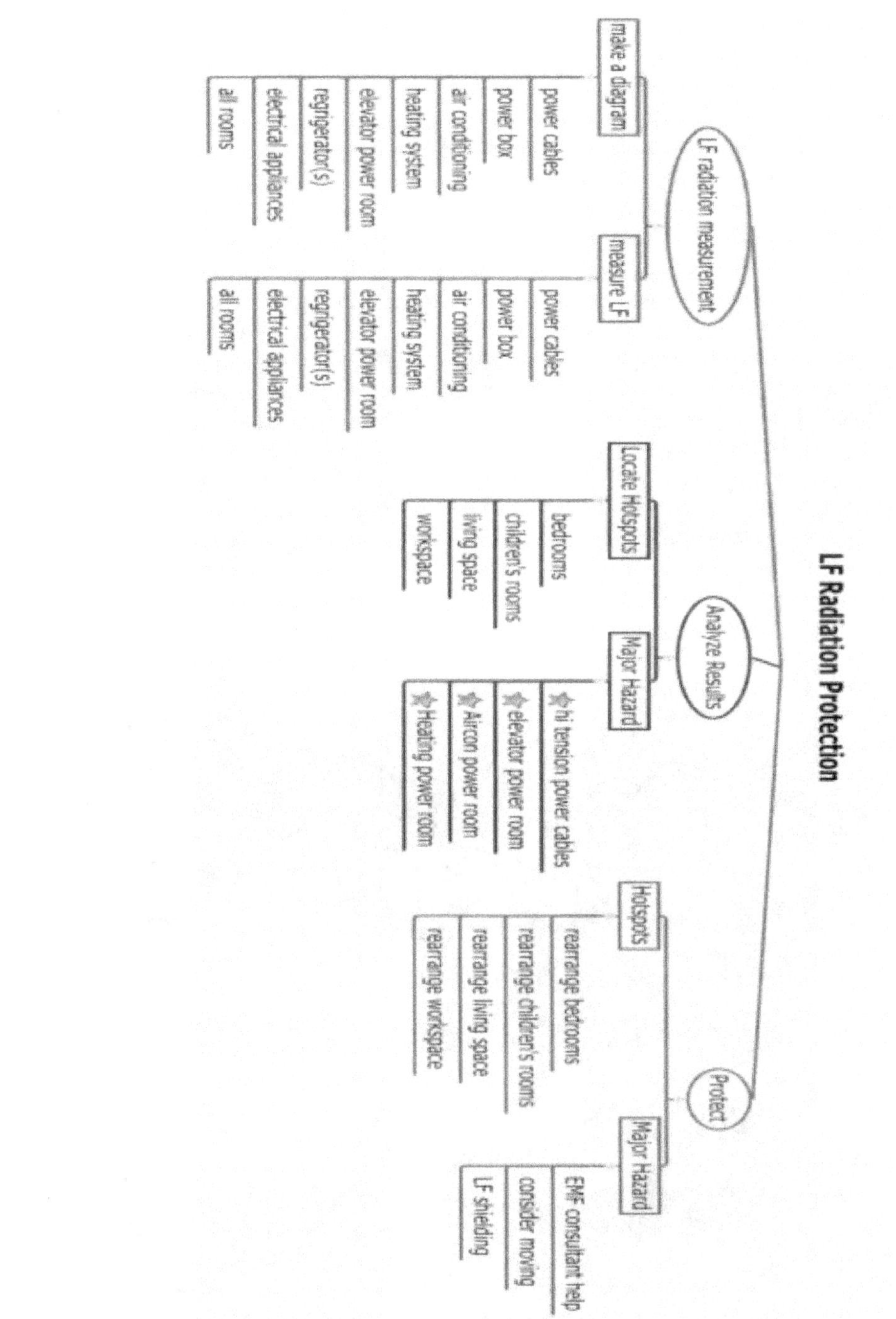
LF Radiation Protection
LF radiation measurement
make a diagram
power cables
power box
air conditioning
heating system
elevator power room
regrigerator(s)
electrical appliances
all rooms
measure LF
power cables
power box
air conditioning
heating system
elevator power room
regrigerator(s)
electrical appliances
all rooms
Analyze Results
Locate Hotspots
bedrooms
children's rooms
living space
workspace
Major Hazard
hi tension power cables
elevator power room
Aircon power room
Heating power room
Protect
Hotspots
rearrange bedrooms
rearrange children's rooms
rearrange living space
rearrange workspace
Major Hazard
EMF consultant help
consider moving
LF shielding

Image 5.1 - LF radiation close to an electric toothbrush (when turned on)

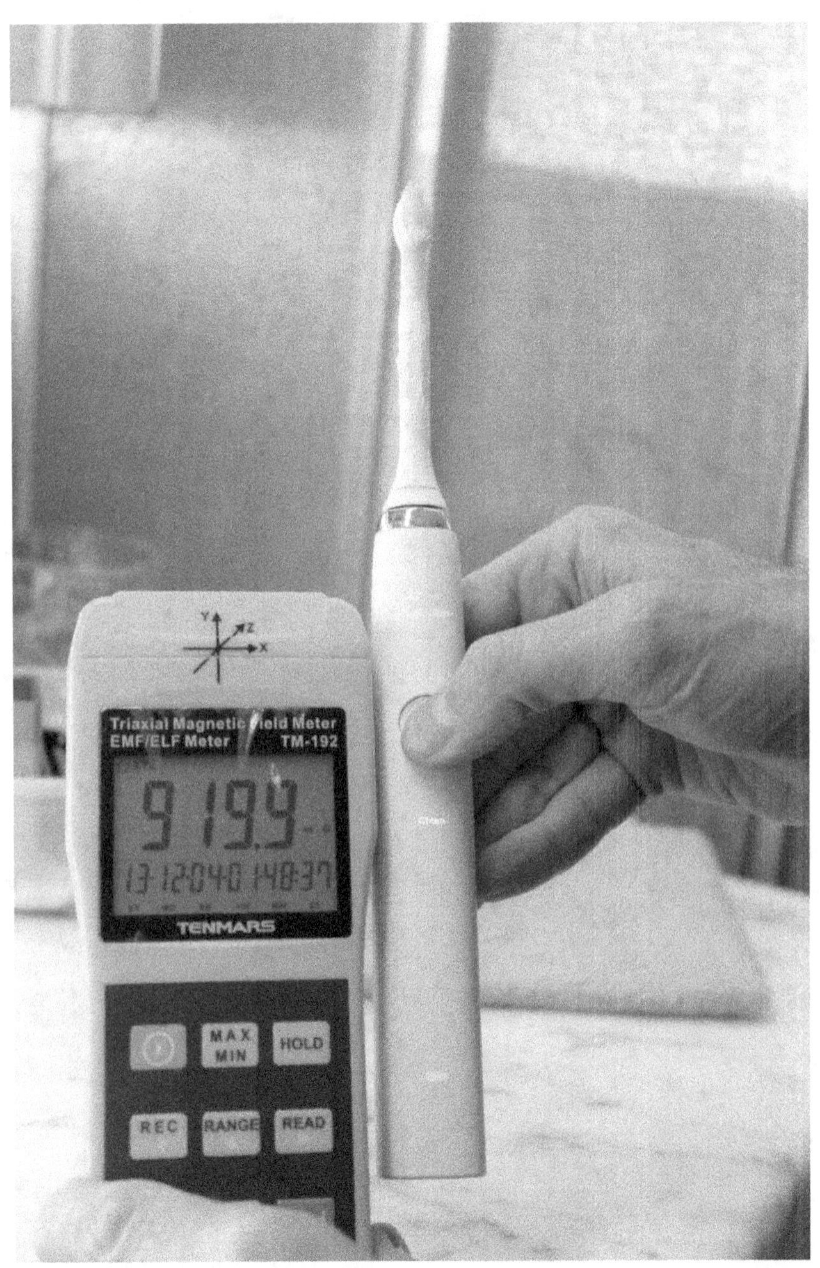

Image 5.2 - LF radiation close to a blender (when turned on)

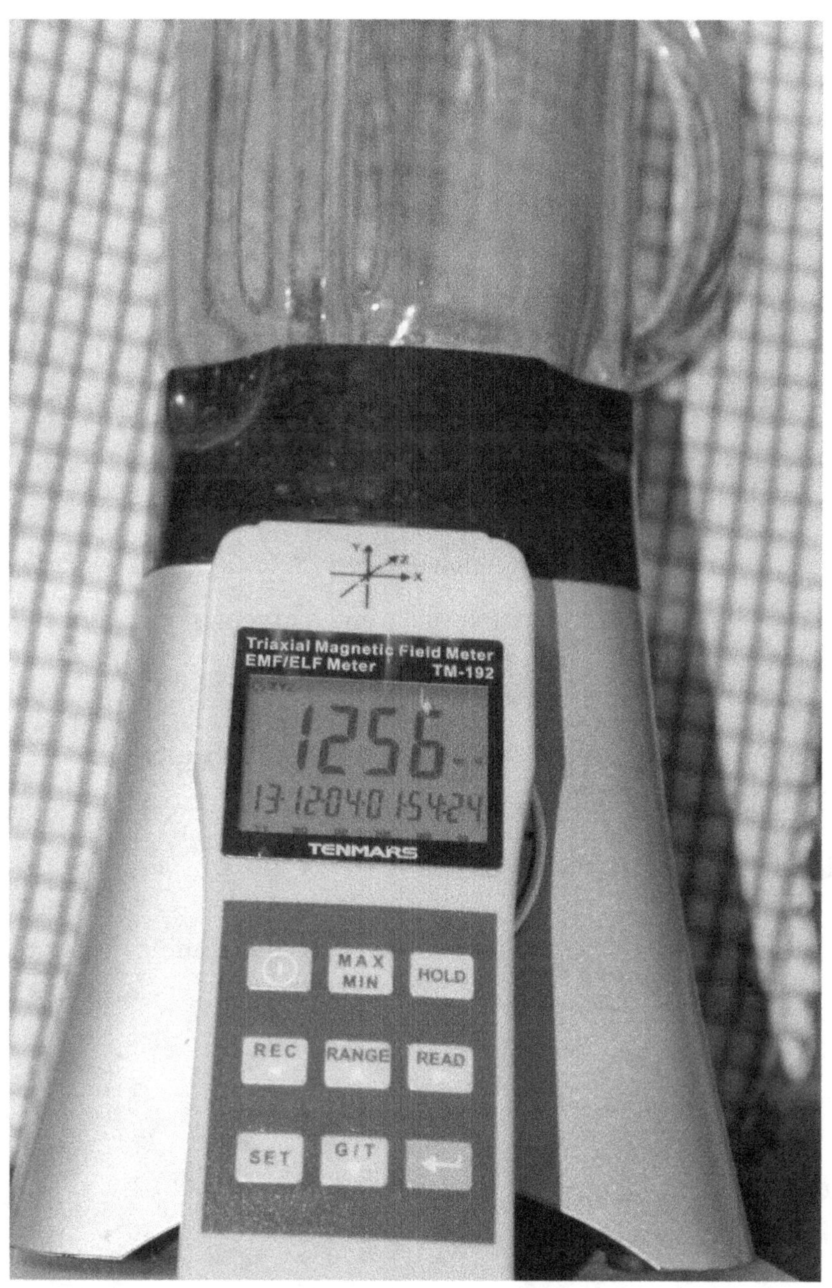

6 DIRTY ELECTRICITY PROTECTION

Assessing levels of dirty electricity

There are two ways to assess levels of dirty electricity in your home's (or office) electrical network. You can use a special oscilloscope that is capable of measuring and analyzing various parameters of your electrical network. However, special scopes are very expensive and designed for professionals. Luckily, there is a much cheaper and simpler solution. It is called a Micro-Surge Meter. This meter has been developed by Prof. Martin Graham from Berkeley University and by Mr. Dave Stetzer. It works by separating high and low frequencies on the power line to detect low level high frequency voltages caused by transients and harmonics. It is very easy to use. To operate the meter, you simply plug it into the power socket and read the display.

The measurement results are given in **GS (Graham-Stetzer) units**. A reading of **50 and above** indicates an unhealthy level of dirty electricity and indicates that you need to take action to correct the situation. Ideally the reading **should be below 30 GS units.**

In many homes the Microsurge meter may show very high readings indicating that the level of dirty electricity is very high.

Image 6.1 Measuring Dirty Electricity

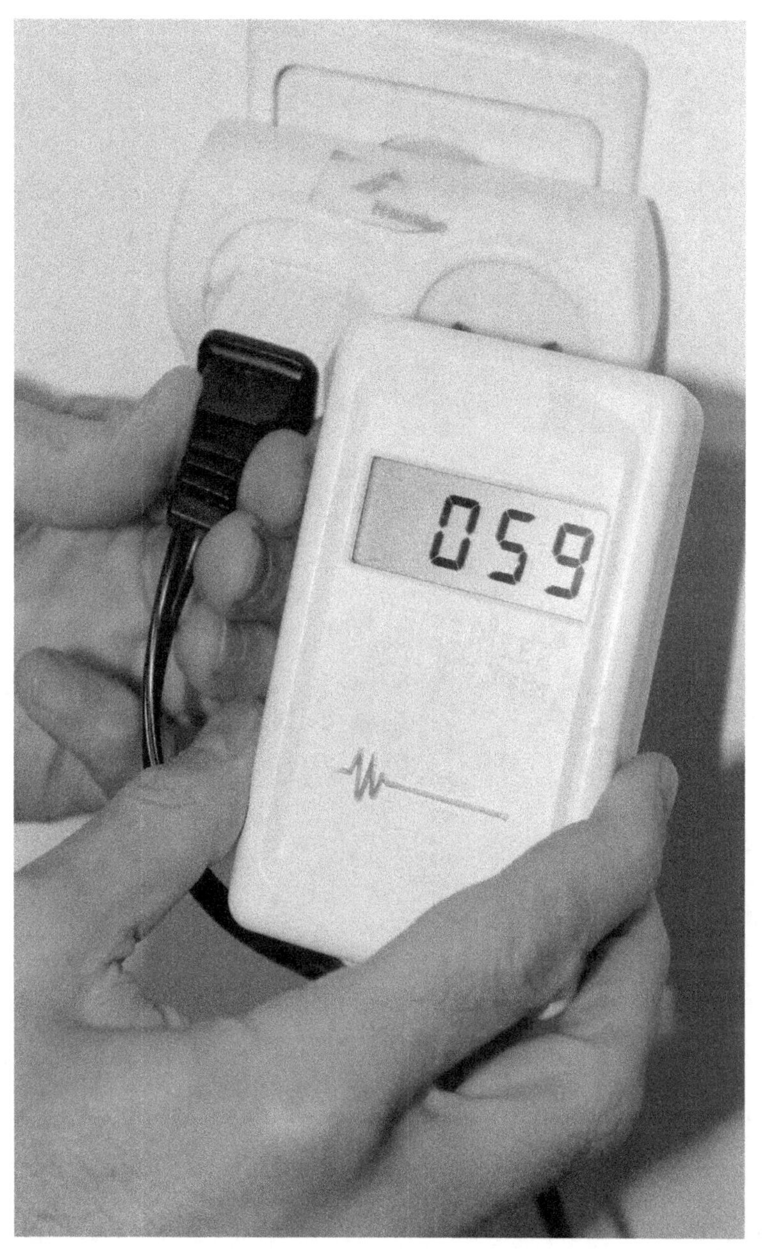

Image 6.2 Measuring again after installing a Micro-Surge Filter

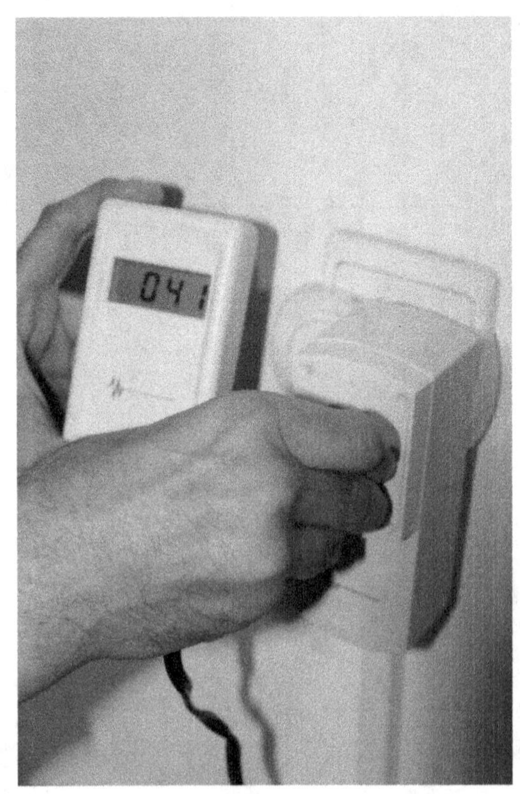

Taking action to reduce dirty electricity

First - identify devices that introduce high levels of dirty electricity and where possible replace them with other devices or disconnect them when not in use. Use a   Dirty Electricity Meter to measure every socket in your house and gradually you will be able to identify trouble spots by disconnecting and reconnecting devices suspected of creating dirty electricity. Many harmless looking electrical components and electronic devices actually produce high levels of dirty electricity. These include dimmer switches, fluorescent lamps, compact fluorescent lamps (CFLs), some (usually poor quality) led lamps, electronic devices and computers. Fluorescent lamps and CFLs save power but they create high levels of dirty electricity, emit high levels of unhealthy UV light and some still contain mercury. They are advertised as "green" but unfortunately this does not always equate with "healthy". Dimmer switches may also help save power and allow more control over light intensity. However, most incorporate electrical circuits that introduce dirty electricity into your electrical network. Led lamps may be very economical. Good quality led lamps do not produce high levels of dirty electricity but lower quality ones may produce significant levels of dirty electricity. The only way to know for sure is to compare the levels of dirty electricity when these components are on and when they are off.

If after taking the necessary steps described above, you still detect high levels of dirty electricity then you may need to install special microsurge filters that allow only low frequency ("clean") electricity to remain in your system by draining out all the high frequency micro-surges. These filters are easy to install. You simply plug them into electrical sockets. You need to install the filters in every room and along every branch of your electrical network, and in particular close to the main power box, and in every socket that supplies power to dirty electricity generating devices (e.g. computers). After plugging the filter into the socket use the Microsurge Meter again to measure the residual level of dirty electricity. Keep working your way through the house until you have reduced levels of dirty electricity to below 50 GS throughout the house. A typical three-bedroom apartment needs about 12 dirty electricity / microsurge filters. A house may require more.

Notes:

1. Use only filters that have been designed and certified for use in your country/ state.

2. Never use filters that have been designed for use in other countries.

3. Follow the manufacturer's instructions carefully.

4. If you are not sure of any of the details in the manufacturer's instructions, get an EMF professional to take dirty electricity readings and install the filters.

Figure 6.1 Dirty Electricity (DE) Protection Strategy

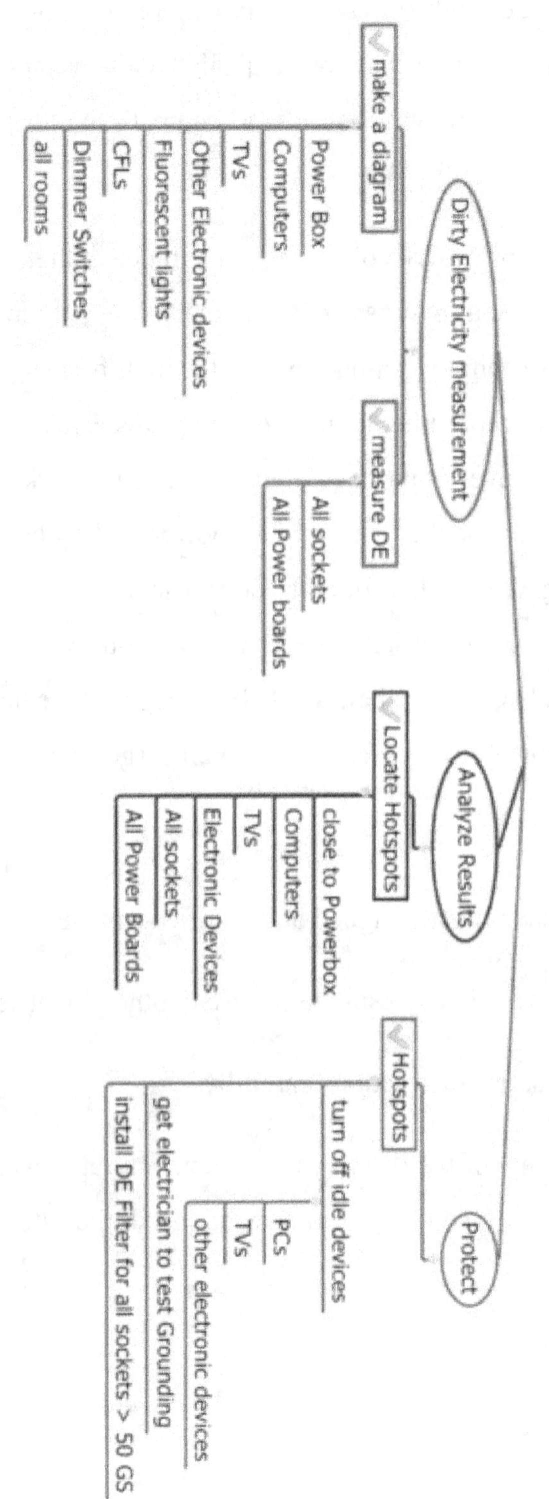

7 RADIO FREQUENCY (RF) PROTECTION

RF electromagnetic fields are all around us

As explained in the introduction we are exposed to diverse RF radiation sources both outdoors and indoors. Most prevalent outdoor sources include cell-phone towers, microwave communication towers, Wi-Max networks, radio and TV transmissions, radar stations. Most prevalent indoor sources include Wi-Fi routers, Wi-Fi enabled devices (e.g. laptops, tablets), DECT phones and cell-phones.

Basic RF protection strategy

In some ways dealing with RF is much easier than dealing with LF because RF radiation is easier to shield. On the other hand, the diversity of RF sources and our growing dependence on mobile technology presents considerable challenges. An effective RF protection strategy requires combining several defensive measures mentioned in previous sections including avoidance, reduction, reflection, absorption as well as making a range of lifestyle modifications. Because of the diversity of RF sources we will describe a range of general and device specific or situation specific RF protection strategies.

Identifying major RF sources in your environment

Before conducting any measurements, you need to make a list of RF sources in your environment as these may affect your choice of RF meter when you buy one.

1. If you are living right next to an FM radio station you may be exposed to significant levels of VHF.

2. If you are living right next to a TV station you may be exposed to significant levels of UHF.

3. If you are living next to a microwave telecommunication tower or cell phone base station you may be exposed to significant levels of UHF and/or SHF radiation.

4. If you spend much time close to a Smart Meter, Wi-Fi router or another source of Wi-Fi transmission then you may be exposed to significant levels of UHF and/or SHF radiation.

5. If you live next to a radar station, then you may be exposed to significant levels of SHF radiation.

6. If you use your cell phone frequently either directly or via a Bluetooth device, then you may be exposed to significant levels of UHF radiation.

7. If you or your neighbors use Wi-Fi at home or at work then you may be exposed to significant levels of UHF radiation.

Measuring Radio Frequency (RF) Radiation

In this section we will explain in detail how to measure radio frequency (RF) electromagnetic radiation. Conducting methodical and accurate RF radiation measurements is an important step you need to take before you can start planning and implementing your RF radiation protection strategy. Measuring RF is by far more complex than measuring ELF electromagnetic fields. There are several reasons for this:

1. The great diversity of RF sources

2. A wide range of RF frequencies

3. Diversity in modes of transmission (constant, variable, pulsing, intermittent etc.)

Getting the right RF meter

Frequency range considerations

In order to measure RF accurately you need to get the right RF meter(s). The information above underlines the need to get a reasonable quality meter that is able to handle all RF sources that may be affecting you. Wi-Fi and cell phone transmissions are gradually being allocated larger chunks of the RF spectrum and some meters may not be able to detect and measure all of these RF transmissions. Some RF meters can only measure up to 2.8 GHZ, 3 GHz or 3.5 GHz. However, there is a new generation of Wi-Fi routers that can also use the 5 GHz band in addition to the older 2.4 GHz band. So as you can see it is better to get a RF meter that can handle a wide range of frequencies. At the time of writing this book you would probably do well to get a meter that can detect and measure up to 8 GHz in order to enable you to measure most present and future RF hazards that may crop up. There are all sorts of RF meters on the market. For self-use there is no need to get a professional level meter as it can be quite expensive. On the other hand, I don't recommend getting a cheap meter as most are of poor quality and may not perform reliably. There are plenty of good meters in the mid-price range.

Single-axis versus Tri-axial RF meters

There are basically two types of RF meters - single axis and tri-axis meters. Single axis directional RF meters and Tri-axial RF meters both have advantages and disadvantages depending on exact meter configuration and design. Here are the main characteristics that set them apart:

1. Single-axis (directional) meters only measure the EMR level along one axis (for example the X axis) whereas tri-axial meters measure the radiation levels along each of the three axes (X, Y and Z) in relation to the meter's orientation at the time of taking a reading. Tri-axial meters also have a built in algorithm that sums up the results from all three axes to approximate the total radiation level.

2. When using single-axis directional meters you need to tilt the meter slowly in different directions until you get the highest reading. This may be time consuming. Tri-axial meters save time during measurement. You get a good idea of the overall and maximum radiation level almost instantly. In most Triaxial meters you can also get a separate reading for each of the three axes (X, Y, Z) just like in a single axis meter.

3. Having said that, some of the best meters are directional. They are typically equipped with a very long logarithmic antenna. By pointing the tip of the antenna and scanning the environment until you get the strongest signal you may be able to detect and pinpoint the direction the RF radiation is coming from or even the actual source. It would be difficult to

achieve this level of precision in detecting the direction the RF is coming from without a logarithmic antenna. Remember, there are diverse sources of RF transmissions all around us. Because RF waves have a much smaller wavelength than LF waves it is possible to shield effectively against RF if (BIG IF) you know the direction the RF radiation is coming from. For example: If you use RF shielding paint to shield the wrong wall then RF radiation levels in your house may actually go up. If there are two sources of RF radiation coming from two different directions and you only shield the wall facing the strongest source, radiation levels inside your house may still increase because radiation coming from the weaker RF source might enter the house from one side, travel through the house and then get reflected back into the house by the shielded wall on the other side. Therefore, it is an advantage to be able to detect, pinpoint and distinguish between different sources of RF radiation in order to shield effectively against all of them. And for this purpose a quality directional RF meter with a logarithmic antenna is much better.

Functions you should look for when buying an EMF meter

1. Several types of units **are** used to measure RF electromagnetic fields:
   - **Electric Field Strength** (E) given in millivolt per meter (mV/m)
   - **Magnetic Field Strength** (H) given in Amperes per meter (A/m)
   - **Power Density** (S) - given in Watts per square meter (W/m2) OR milliwatt per square centimeter (mW/cm^2) or micro-Watt per square centimeter (µW/cm2). Power density represents the power per unit area normal to the direction of propagation of the electromagnetic field. This is the most commonly used unit to measure RF radiation coming from a distance. This is the unit you will most often encounter in various reports and articles, including the Bioinitiative report. So you would probably be using Power Density units in most of your measurements.

2. Another useful feature is the **MAX/MIN** function. This function allows determining minimum and maximum radiation levels within a specified time frame. It is especially important to be able to determine maximum value if the RF field intensity fluctuates constantly (e.g. in Wi-Fi routers).

3. Another useful feature is the **AVG** function. This function allows determining average radiation levels within a specified time frame. It is especially important to be able to determine average value if the RF field intensity fluctuates constantly (e.g. in Wi-Fi routers).

4. Another useful function is the **HOLD** function that freezes the value on the display and enables you to write it down.

5. Another useful function is the **Record** function that enables you to store results in the meter's memory and retrieve them later.

6. Another useful function allows recording values over a specified **TIME** frame. This allows sampling and recording radiation levels over minutes or hours. You can leave the meter on and it will record and store the data automatically over time allowing you to analyze it later and get a better picture of radiation fluctuations, **MIN, MAX and AVG** over time.

7. An important function is **Auto shut-down**. This function can be set to shut down the meter if it is inactive for a pre-set length of time. This will significantly extend the life of the battery.

Making a diagram of the house, apartment or office

Before you start measuring, prepare a sketch of your apartment or house. A simple sketch will do. The sketch needs to include the following elements:

1. Location of cell-phone towers in relation to your house

2. Location of microwave transmission towers in relation to your house

3. Location of radio and TV stations in relation to your house

4. Location of Smart Meters outside your house and outside neighbors' houses

5. Location of Wi-Fi router inside your house or apartment

6. Location of Wi-Fi routers in your neighbors' houses or apartments

7. Locations of DECT phone base station in your house or apartment

8. Locations of DECT phone base station in your neighbors' houses or apartments

Taking RF radiation measurements in each of the rooms

Levels of RF radiation may vary considerably within a single room. Therefore, you need to take several measurements in each room. As a minimum I suggest that you perform the following measurements:

1. Measure radiation levels next to the each of the windows

2. Measure radiation levels in each of the beds where people normally sleep

3. Measure radiation levels in the children's play areas

4. Measure radiation levels in each of the armchairs and sofas where you spend time relaxing

5. Measure radiation levels around your work desk

6. Measure radiation levels in each of the four corners of each room, next to the wall halfway between the two corners and at the center of each room.

7. Measure radiation levels next to your Wi-Fi router

8. Measure radiation levels in each of the rooms when the Wi-Fi router is on and when it is off to get an idea of the effect of the Wi-Fi router on radiation levels throughout your house. I recommended always disabling the router's Wi-Fi functionality and using Ethernet cables to connect computers and laptops to the router.

9. Some routers restart their Wi-Fi broadcasts after rebooting and after a power failure. Some even restart their Wi-Fi automatically after downloading an automatic update via the Internet. This is a real pain. It is impossible to keep up with all these changes. There are solutions to this annoying problem. The most obvious solution is to purchase a router that does not have a Wi-Fi feature at all. Another solution is to shop around for a router that has a Wi-Fi button on the front panel that allows turning the Wi-Fi off at will. Verify with the vendor and manufacturer that the Wi-Fi will stay off unless you turn it on again by pressing

the Wi-Fi button. Don't settle for less because you may unknowingly be spending much time next to a powerful source of RF radiation.

10. Measure radiation levels next to the smart meter outside your house and inside the house close to the wall where the Smart meter was installed (on the other side). You may need to set the RF meter to record for a few minutes or even a few hours to determine how frequently the smart meter is really transmitting. You may be unpleasantly surprised to find out that the smart meter is transmitting every minute or two and not several times a day as advertised in some cases.

11. Measure radiation levels next to the baby's wireless remote monitor. You may be unpleasantly surprised to find out that the monitor is emitting substantial RF radiation. I suggest you try to find and install a wired baby monitor if it is available as babies are much more sensitive and vulnerable to electromagnetic radiation than adults. The section on Baby EMF protection strategies discusses this in detail.

Analyzing measurement results

1. Before we start analyzing our measurement results let's remind ourselves of the recommended safety limits:

   The 2012 Bioinitiative Report recommended **a precautionary level** of between $0.0003 \ \mu W/cm^2$ to $0.0006 \ \mu W/cm^2$. For outdoor RF radiation exposure, the 2007 Bioinitiative Report recommended a limit of $0.1 \ \mu W/cm^2$.

2. If you only detect RF hot-spots, in other words you do not detect an overall high level of RF in your house or office then you can probably work around the hot-spots and protect yourself effectively against RF.

3. If on the other hand, significant portions of your house or office have high levels of RF radiation this is not a good sign. The source may be a cell phone tower, a microwave communication tower, a TV or radio station or a radar station close by. The source may also be a powerful Wi-Fi system installed in the building or a powerful Wi-Max system installed outside the building.

4. The good news - unlike LF radiation, RF radiation can be shielded quite effectively. However, if a powerful RF source is close by then shielding your entire house may be expensive and require significant work. Also, even if you totally shield your house from all directions, you will still be exposed to high levels of RF radiation when you spend time in your backyard or go for a walk around the block. In such cases you may consider relocation.

Dealing with RF hotspots

1. If you have only detected RF hot-spots inside your house, apartment or office then you may be able to deal with them quite effectively. Here are the main steps you need to take:

2. If the RF radiation is coming from a relatively distant cell phone tower or communication tower, you need to shield the windows and walls facing in that direction. Shield the walls with RF shielding paint. Shield the windows with transparent RF shielding film and with RF shielding curtains. If the radiation is also coming through the roof you may need to paint the ceiling with RF shielding paint. You may consider installing a double layer of aluminum foil insulation under the roof.

3. If you find an RF hot-spot created by your Wi-Fi router I recommended you disable the router's Wi-Fi functionality and connect your computers to the router via an Ethernet cable.

4. If you find an RF hot-spot created by your DECT phone I recommended you get an old fashioned phone or phone(s) and install them in convenient places. DECT phones and their base stations emit very high radiation levels.

5. If you find an RF hot spot created by a Smart Meter installed outside your house, try to have the meter replaced by a regular meter. If that is not possible you can block the meter's radiation by painting the inside wall with RF shielding paint.

6. If the RF radiation is coming from Wi-Fi routers in neighboring apartments try to identify the exact location. If you are on friendly terms with your neighbors, you can ask them where the router is located and then you can block the router's radiation by painting the adjoining wall inside your apartment with RF shielding paint.

7. If you are still not happy with RF levels in your bedroom you can hang an RF shielding canopy over your bed.

RF radiation Protection for Windows, Doors and other Openings

It is important to understand that a substantial amount of RF radiation penetrates your home or office via windows and doors. Solid walls made of brick, steel and stone absorb significant percent of RF radiation, especially in the millimeter bandwidth. However, windows made of glass or synthetic materials are transparent not only to light but also to electromagnetic waves. Wooden doors are also transparent to electromagnetic waves, whereas steel doors may reflect most RF waves that hit them. Therefore, the first step in protecting a room against an external source of RF radiation is to secure any windows and external doors. After you have secured all windows and doors, re-measure RF EMR levels. Only if they are still too high, consider using RF shielding paints for other RF shielding materials on the wall(s)

RF Protection methods for windows

You may choose a combination of the following methods to protect your windows against RF radiation

1. **Installing a metallic mesh fly screen**

   This is by far the cheapest method. The screen serves a double purpose as it also keeps out flies. However, in some windows a sliding fly screen only covers half the width of the window. Metallic fly screens are actually a wire mesh made of aluminium, galvanized iron, copper or stainless steel. The copper has the best EMR shielding properties but others will do. Buy several small samples first and test them at home on one window to see which works better for you. You can further improve RF shielding by using a double layer of the wire mesh. The more layers the better the shielding effect. After installing the fly screen re-measure radiation levels to determine if you need to take further protective measures.

2. **Installing an RF shielding curtain**

   You can buy a good quality RF shielding fabric and make your own curtain. Make sure the curtain's width and height are both at least a meter longer than the window frame's width and height respectively to make sure radiation does not penetrate around the corners. RF shielding curtains provide better protection than the metallic fly screen because they are made of materials that have better RF reflection properties and also because you can make them wider and taller than the window frame. However, RF shielding curtains only reflect RF when they are fully drawn. If you draw the curtain aside to let more light or air in you immediately lose your RF protection.

3. **Installing RF shielding transparent sheets or films**

   Another method that you can use to shield against RF radiation coming through the window is to apply a transparent sheet or transparent film on the window panes. These can provide good RF shielding properties as long as the window is shut. Combining this method with an RF shielding curtain and a metallic fly net gives the best results.

RF Protection methods for doors

Doors are easier to shield than windows. Some doors that are made of metal may reflect a significant percentage of RF radiation. Here are some effective ways to make your doors RF safe:

1. Paint the door with RF shielding paint and then apply several top coats. The problem with this method is that it is very difficult to ground the door. Still, you may achieve some level of relatively inexpensive RF protection

2. Glue RF shielding fabric or RF shielding wallpaper on the inside of the door. Choose a fabric that is easy to work with and that is easy to glue on the door's inner surface. Cut holes for door knobs, key holes

3. If you have a screen door make sure the screen is made from metallic mesh. If not, then change the mesh to a metallic mesh with good RF reflective properties.

Using RF shielding paints

RF shielding paints are an essential component of EMF radiation protection. To use RF shielding paints effectively you need to make sure that the overall level of radiation in all bandwidths decreases in other words you need to make sure that you are not creating a second problem while solving the first. Remember:

1. **Effective RF protection requires both technological and behavioral counter measures.**

2. **Applying only technological measures may not be enough and in some cases may prove to be counterproductive.**

3. **Applying effective RF shielding measures requires basic understanding how the technology works.**

How do RF shielding paints work?

RF shielding paints work mostly by reflecting RF radiation (bouncing it back the same as a mirror reflects light). For example, a typical RF shielding paint may reflect 85 to 88 percent of the radiation, absorb up to 10 percent and allow 2 to 5 percent to go through, thus providing a total of 95 to 98 percent reduction in EMR (electromagnetic radiation).

Basic RF shielding paint decisions

There are several basic decisions you need to make when selecting and applying RF shielding paint. The choices you make will depend on the location and magnitude of RF source and also on the area you are shielding. Here are some questions you need to ask yourself before making a decision:

1. Do I use the paint on the external or internal side of the wall?

2. Do I apply the paint all the way up to the ceiling?

3. Do I apply the paint to the ceiling as well?

4. Do I apply the paint to one wall or several walls?

5. Do I need to ground the paint?

6. Which paint do I choose?

The answers to these questions will determine how you proceed. There are no clear cut answers and your final decision will probably be based on optimizing several deciding factors. Here are some points that will help you reach an optimal solution:

1. RF shielding paints are rather expensive so you want to protect the RF paint and keep it intact for a long time. After applying the RF shielding paint you need to apply a top coat over it. The top coast consists of several layers of ordinary paint. Under normal conditions the top coat is enough to protect your RF shielding paint. However, if the external walls are exposed to harsh weather conditions you may consider applying your RF shielding paint on the internal side of the wall and not the external side. Harsh weather conditions include extreme temperature differences between day and night, high humidity or extreme dryness, strong winds, heavy rains and snows.

2. Under normal conditions external walls require more paint than internal walls, for example 1 litre of RF shielding paint may allow covering 7.5 square meters on an internal wall but only 5 square meters on an external wall. If the external walls are very weather-worn, rough, flaking or chapped they would probably require even more RF shielding paint in order to get a uniform and adequate protective shield. If your external walls are in very poor condition, you may consider applying your RF shielding paint on internal and not on external walls.

3. If your walls are thick and solid (e.g. concrete and steel or stone walls), and if the external side of the walls is relatively smooth and if weather conditions are reasonably mild, then you should consider applying your RF shielding paint on the external side of the walls. One important reason for doing this would be a scenario of two sources of EMR coming from two different directions. For example, a major source of EMR on the east and a minor source of EMR on the west. Thick walls are able to absorb a significant percentage of RF radiation. If radiation only comes from one direction, then you can block it effectively by applying the RF shielding paint either to the internal or external side of the wall. However, if a main source of RF radiation is located on one side of the house (e.g. the east) and a secondary weaker source of RF radiation is located on the opposite side (e.g. the west), then applying RF shielding paint on the internal side of a wall may yield undesirable

results. You may block the radiation coming from the main RF source (from the east) effectively. However, the radiation coming from the secondary RF source (from the west in this example) would travel through the house until it reaches the RF shielding paint on the other side of the house and most of it would then be reflected back into the house. This would create an interesting situation because radiation coming from the secondary RF source would travel twice through the house and effectively radiation exposure from this source would be doubled. If you encounter a similar situation it would be better to paint the external side of the eastern facing wall because most of the secondary radiation coming from the west would be absorbed by the wall before reaching the external RF shielding paint and the reflection of the secondary RF source back into the house would be minimal. At this point you are probably asking yourself: Why not solve the problem by painting the internal side of both eastern and western facing walls. And of course this would be the ideal solution. However, it would also be more expensive and labor intensive.

4. Some RF shielding paints are mostly suitable for internal walls. Some are suitable for both external and internal walls. Some RF shielding paints have very good weather resistance properties and some do not. Make sure you get the right paint for the solution you have chosen.

Basic RF Paint application procedure

I am not going to get into too much detail on this topic simply because RF shielding paints come with instructions provided by the manufacturer. To get the best results you need to follow these instructions. Furthermore, most RF shielding paints require grounding and that should ONLY be done by a qualified electrician. This section is not intended as a substitute for professional help. The purpose of this section is only to give you a general idea of the main steps that are usually taken when applying a typical RF shielding paint application checklist. Some of the steps may vary depending on the house's specific circumstances and manufacturer's instructions.

CAUTION: NEVER attempt any electrical and grounding work yourself. Electricity is dangerous. Electrical work done by unqualified people may lead to electrocution, physical injury or even death.

Here is a typical RF shielding paint application sequence

1. Decide which wall(s) need RF protection

2. Decide whether to apply the RF paint on the internal or external side of the wall. There are different grounding kits for internal and external walls. Make sure you order the grounding kit suitable for the solution you have chosen.

3. Prepare the wall surface for painting

4. **Get a qualified electrician to test the grounding and install the necessary grounding connections.** Electrical grounding is very important and can save lives. If your house or apartment does not have electrical grounding you need to get a qualified electrician to assess the situation. Ideally the electrician would be able to add grounding to your electrical network. However, in cases where this is not possible or applicable, the electrician may be able to provide a separate grounding solution for the RF shielding paint.
    The electrician needs to test and decide whether or not the RF shielding paint will be grounded via the house grounding. If house' grounding does not exist or is not suitable – then the electrician needs to consider other grounding options (e.g. using an external grounding rod) These options can only be applied by a qualified electrician who has all the necessary testing equipment.
    NOTE: Electricity can be dangerous and may lead to electrocution, physical injury or even death. Any electrical work should only be performed by a qualified electrician.

5. The electrician needs to apply the horizontal and vertical conductive tapes along the wall(s) following manufacturer's instructions while making sure the tapes are well away from any electrical sockets.

6. Some RF shielding paint may have to be applied to a small area of the wall before the electrician can mount the grounding plate on it. Ask the electrician where to paint the wall with RF paint.

7. The electrician needs to mount the grounding plate on the wall and connect it to the house'
grounding or to an external grounding solution as per manufacturer's instructions. The
electrician needs to choose the area for mounting the grounding plate carefully to make
sure no electrical wires are present.

CAUTION: DO NOT attempt doing it yourself. Only a qualified electrician with suitable
testing equipment should do this

8. After all, grounding connections are in place the electrician needs to test to test grounding
quality and verify that no electrical shorts exist. This is extremely important because RF
shielding paint is electrically conductive and wrong application of the grounding may lead
to walls conducting electrical currents!!!

CAUTION: Never attempt doing any electrical and grounding work yourself. Electricity is
dangerous. Electrical work done by unqualified people may lead to electrocution, physical
injury or even death.

Behavioral modifications related to application of shielding paints

RF shielding paints are an important and very effective tool to protect against RF RMR. However,
without proper understanding and behavioral modifications, RF shielding paints may become a
double edged sword that solves one problem and creates another.

To illustrate why behavioral modifications are required after applying RF shielding paints let's
look at the following scenario. Let's say that you want to protect your apartment from an external
source of RF microwave radiation such as a cell phone base station or a telecommunication tower.
Let's say that you have identified the location of the RF source, measured RF radiation levels
inside and outside your house, selected the wall(s) for applying RF shielding paint, applied the RF
shielding paint and grounded it following the manufacturer's instructions with the help of a
qualified electrician as mentioned above.

After having applied all the measures described above you may think that you have completely
solved your RF radiation problem. However, this may prove to be a false assumption unless you
have also implemented behavioral and lifestyle changes. The reflective property of the RF
shielding paint may actually increase levels of EMF in the shielded room if you continue to use

your Wi-Fi router, Wi-Fi enabled devices, DECT phones and mobile phones inside your apartment or house. Why is that? Because some of the radiation generated by the Wi-Fi router or mobile phone, which would normally exit via the wall would now be reflected back into the house by the RF shielding paint. To eliminate this problem, you need to make the necessary behavioral and lifestyle changes! In this particular example it means that you need to disable your router's Wi-Fi functionality and connect the computer to the router using an Ethernet cable as discussed in detail in a previous section. Furthermore, you need to avoid as much as possible using your cell-phone inside the apartment. You also need to stop using your DECT phones and use a wired phone instead.

CAUTION:

1. You should not attempt to do any electrical work by yourself as this can be dangerous, may lead to electrocution or even death.

2. Shielding paints may require grounding. Grounding should only be installed by a qualified electrician following manufacturer's instructions.

Image 7.1 - RF Radiation of an operating Microwave Oven

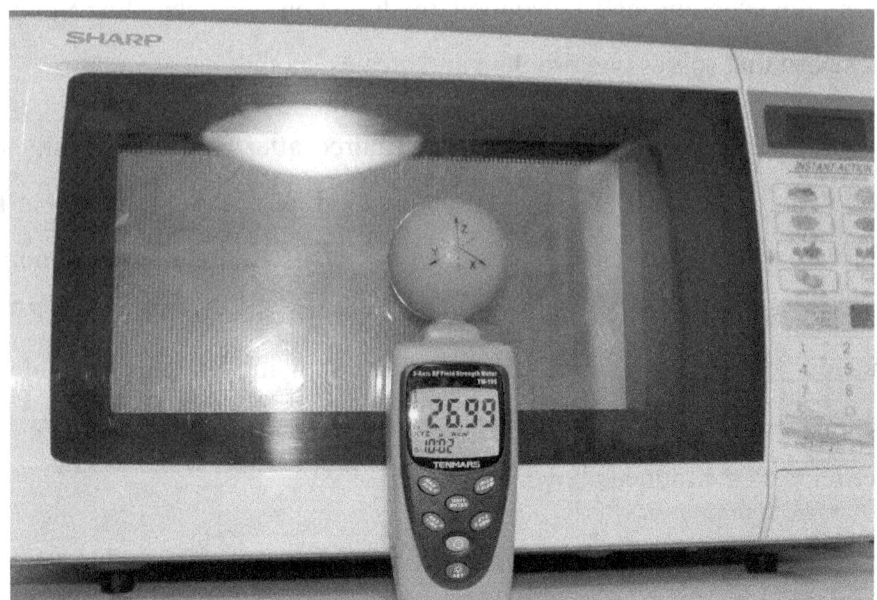

Figure 7.1 - RF Radiation Protection Strategy

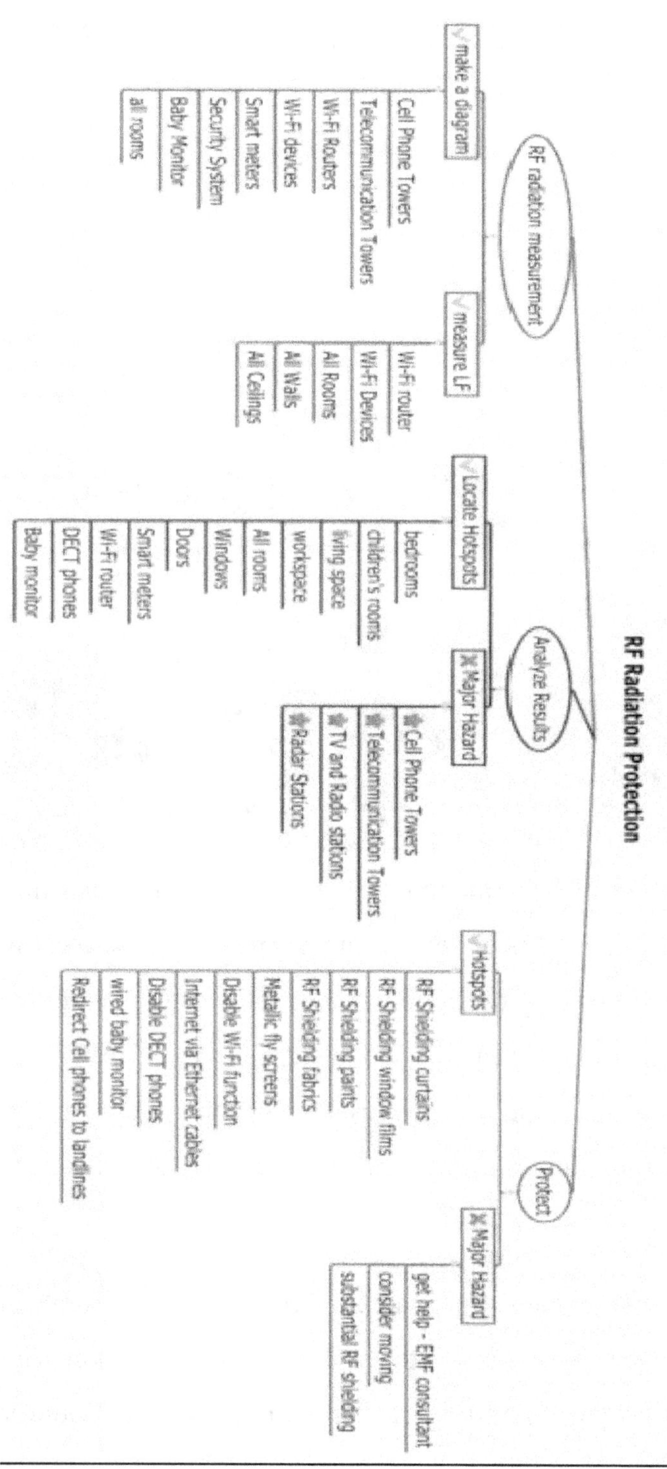

8 CELL PHONE EMF PROTECTION

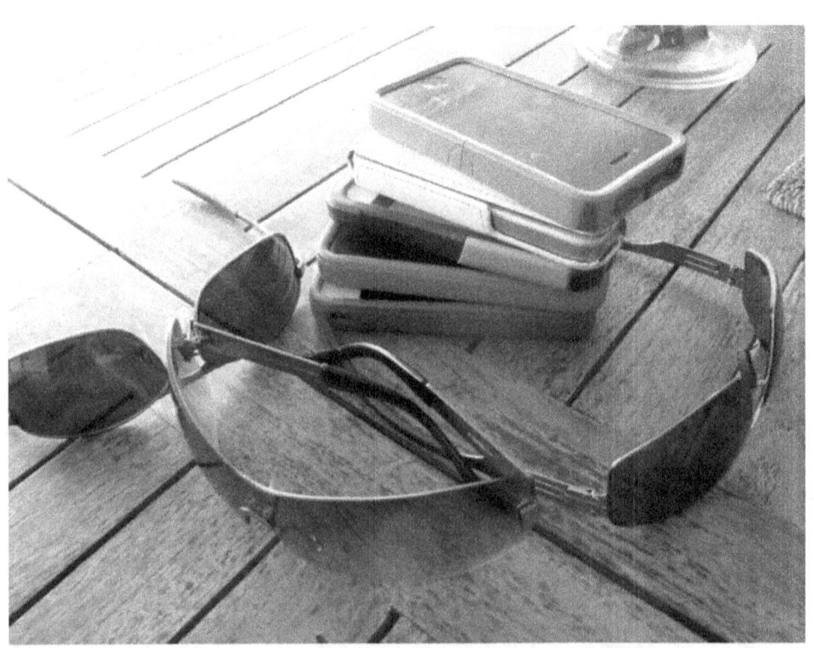

One of the major sources of RF radiation in our lives is the growing number of cell-phones. Cell phones, also called mobile phones or cellular phones have become one of the most commonly used devices today. The cell-phone subscription rate in the western world is almost 100% and in the developing countries it is moving rapidly in the same direction. As a matter of fact, in developing countries with poor infrastructure, cell phones have become the main form of telecommunication. Cell phones have become universal affecting people from all walks of life and socio-economic backgrounds.

Unfortunately, as the saying goes - 'there are no free lunches'. The price that we pay for using cell-phones is an ever increasing exposure to electromagnetic radiation (EMR) that affects all cell phone users and also people who are in close proximity (although to a lesser extent). Legislators around the world are making an effort to protect the population from passive smoking in public places but it may take years before the same principle is applied to EMR.

Electromagnetic radiation caused directly and indirectly by cell phones has become a major issue in the area of EMF and health. There are several factors why health risks associated with cell phones have become such a hot issue:

1. The use of cell phones has increased dramatically with the introduction of Smartphones. Smartphones can now be used for any type of Internet activity as well. As a result, exponentially increasing levels of data are being transmitted to and from cell phones. The faster the networks and the more data being transmitted over these networks, the more electromagnetic energy must be transmitted into the environment. Cell phone telecommunication companies are striving to provide the best service they can in order to stay competitive. This means that they are constantly raising the levels of energy emitted from the cell phone towers, in order to overcome obstacles such as roofs and walls in buildings and vehicles. This leads to a rapid increase in electromagnetic energy densities and EMR exposure.

2. Cell phones require cell phone tower base stations and relay stations to be built wherever cell phone reception is required – in other words- everywhere. You can limit your EMR exposure by not using a cell phone but as long as you live in proximity to cell phone towers you are constantly bombarded with EMR whether you like it or not.

3. Telecommunication corporations are lobbying governments to increase allowable maximum electromagnetic radiation levels. Existing safety standards are backed by outdated research. Most recent research has been funded by industry. It is interesting to note that the majority of independent studies have concluded that cell-phone use is associated with increased risk of cancer and a range of other diseases and disorders.

4. Lots of people have become aware of the growing EMF problem and are trying to reduce the time they spend talking on their mobile phones. However, cell phones transmit signals (i.e. emit radiation) even when they are not being used. The reason they do this is to communicate with the cell phone towers to ensure they are always connected to the closest

tower with the strongest signal. People carry their cell-phones with them all day long, and even if they hardly talk, they still absorb a significant cumulative amount of electromagnetic energy.

5. Smartphones also serve as an end point for a range of Internet services and these programs are continuously connecting to the Internet in order to receive messages and updates resulting in frequent transmissions and more radiation.

Is there a way to use the cell phone safely?

The answer is YES and NO. Yes - because there are very effective ways to significantly reduce your exposure to electromagnetic radiation emitted by cell phones. NO - because there is no way to completely eliminate all radiation. Furthermore, some methods claiming to reduce EMR are inherently flawed and may lead to false confidence and higher exposure as explained below.

Cell phones electromagnetic radiation

Cell phones actually emit two types of electromagnetic radiation: Radio frequency (RF) radiation and low frequency (LF) radiation. Most of the energy emitted by cell phones is RF radiation. These frequencies are used by cell-phones to communicate with cell-phone towers and transmit/receive data. LF radiation is a by-product of the phone's internal circuitry, on-board computer, display and speakers. In cell phones LF radiation levels are much lower than RF radiation levels, although not negligible.

Cell phone radiation Protection starts here

In order to protect yourself effectively from cell phone radiation you need to take a range of measures. Before we get into details let us state the four essential mind-set principles that are required to ensure success:

Clear understanding - Gain a clear understanding of EMF/EMR related health risks, how and when radiation is being emitted and the tools available for reducing your exposure. Clear understanding will be the foundation underpinning your cell-phone radiation protection strategy. It will help you make wise choices, increase your level of awareness and vigilance and boost your motivation to overcome temporary inconveniences and entrenched old habits.

Self-discipline - You must exercise self-discipline and stick to your EMR self defence strategy. You must resist temptations and convenient shortcuts. Modern lifestyle has become very fast paced and information driven. Reaching out to a mobile device to check what's new or update others has become second nature to most of us. We need to retrain ourselves to a point where information technology is our servant and we are the masters and not the other way round.

Perseverance - To make a lasting change you need to persevere until you have firmly secured good habits in place. These habits will become part of your new way of life in which you are in control of your health.

Adaptability and flexibility- Stay informed. Join groups of like-minded people. Stay up to date and apply new EMR protection technologies to help you reduce your EMR exposure.

OK, enough theory! Let's roll our sleeves and get to work! Hopefully after applying the following steps your EMR exposure levels will have dropped dramatically making you safer, healthier and hopefully happier.

Cell phone radiation protection strategy

Reduce your cell phone radiation exposure by following these guidelines:

1. Use your cell phone only when you really have to (e.g. for emergencies). If you must use the cell phone keep the conversation short. Better still, if possible use SMS instead of talking. Radiation exposure from sending SMS is only a fraction of radiation exposure while talking on the cell phone. Furthermore, when you SMS the cell-phone is further away from your head (and brain).

2. Try to plan ahead and use other modes of communication wherever they are available. Use land-lines, Skype and similar VOIP (voice over IP) on your computer. Connect your computer via Ethernet cables and not via Wi-Fi. If possible, make use of mail-pigeons (JUST KIDDING!!!)

3. The radiation transmitted from the cell phone's antenna propagates in all directions. As

it spreads it covers a wider area. Consequently, its radiation density decreases in proportion to the square of the distance from the antenna. What this means is that if your cell phone is 1 centimeter away - you absorb up to 10,000 times more radiation than if it is 1 meter away from you! So this clearly demonstrates the need to keep the mobile phone as far as possible from any part of your body, especially from vital organs. The following methods will help you increase the distance between you and the phone when you are using it.

4. Use an air-tube headset (with a long air-tube) in order to keep the radiation away from your head. An air-tube headset terminates in 30 to 50 cm of flexible plastic tube that connects to the earpiece. The plastic tube conducts sound but does not conduct electromagnetic radiation so it keeps the radiation away from your head. Poor quality air-tube headsets provide poor quality sound and tend to fall apart quickly. So I recommend getting a good quality air-tube headset.

5. Get a headset extension cord. Plug the male jack into the phone. Plug the air-tube headset into the female side of the extension cord. When talking position, the phone top of a desk or chair and stand as far away from it as the combined length of the extension cord and air-tube headset allows. This will significantly increase the distance between you and the phone and dramatically reduce your radiation exposure.

6. For home or office use you can use a cell-phone stand/base with a regular handset. Mount your cell-phone in the stand/base and take the call with the phone as far away from you as the handset cord will allow. This is another way to increase the distance between you and the phone without using an air-tube headset.

7. A similar method for home use is to use a cell-phone stand/base/dock that has a powerful speaker and microphone. Mount your cell-phone in the stand/base and take the call with the phone as far away from you as the quality of the speaker and microphone of the base will allow. This is also a way to achieve a substantial distance between you and the phone without using a headset However, it may not be a good way to conduct a private conversation and it may also disturb other people.

8. In an emergency or if you have misplaced your air-tube headset use your cell phone's speaker. Never put the phone next to your head.

9. Using a regular headset is preferable to putting the phone next to your head. A regular headset reduces radiation exposure but an air-tube headset reduces radiation exposure much better. Regular headsets act as a conductor and transfer some of the radiation to your head. They vary in the amount of radiation they conduct and unless you have measured it using an RF meter you will not be able to know exactly what your level of exposure is when using one of these. So I strongly recommend getting a good quality air-tube headset.

10. When your cell phone is in the process of establishing a connection with the other party it emits very high levels of radiation. You are better off waiting until the connection has been made (i.e. the other side picks up and answers) before bringing it closer to your head or body. It only takes a few seconds for radiation levels to drop significantly. So first, make sure your air-tube headset is connected or your speaker phone is on. Then dial keeping the phone as far away from you as possible and when the call has been answered you can bring it closer to you.

11. Follow this procedure when your cell phone rings: Click to reply, keep the phone away from your head and say loudly *"I will be with you in just a second!"* At the same time plug your headset jack or switch to speaker mode. Do not feel bad or embarrassed about it because your number one priority should be to be EMF safe and stay healthy.

12. You can connect to phones directly from your computer using a free Skype account. After you add credit to your Skype credit balance you can use" Skype out" to dial to any phone number from any computer that has Skype installed on it. Connect your computer via Ethernet cables and not via Wi-Fi.

13. Avoid using your cell phone in areas where the reception is poor. You can tell how good the reception is by the number of bars on the phone's reception indicator. In areas with poor reception your cell-phone emits much higher levels of radiation. A Smartphone may emit up to 1000 times more radiation to compensate for poor

reception!!! You may encounter poor reception conditions in some buildings (and not others), in elevators and in basements. The reception inside trains and buses may also be poor because their metal alloy structure reflects and blocks electromagnetic waves. In some rural areas there are very poor reception conditions because cell phone towers are few and far apart. So the country may be a great place to live but not a good place to use the mobile phone safely.

14. If you happen to be located in a building with very poor reception find out if there is a Wi-Fi service available (some may even be free). Try to connect with your Smartphone or tablet to the Internet via the Wi-Fi and then use your "Skype out" to call the phone number you need to connect to. The radiation levels your Smartphone or tablet emit when connecting to a local Wi-Fi service may be much lower than when connecting to the cell phone tower.

15. Avoid using your cell phone inside cars. The cars' metallic body reflects much of the radiation causing it to bounce back and forth inside the vehicle. This significantly increases your radiation exposure. If you must use the phone inside a car -use a hands-free car kit. If you find yourself using the hands-free car kit often, you may consider installing an external antenna on your car's roof. The antenna will keep much of the radiation outside the car and away from you.

16. When at home or at the office divert all your incoming calls to a land-line. Turn the cell-phone off or switch it to air-plane mode when you are not using it.

17. If you do not have access to a landline but do have access to a computer linked to the Internet, divert incoming calls to Skype or similar V.O.I.P. (voice over IP) programs. You may consider getting a Skype number and then you can divert the incoming calls to that number. These calls can in turn be forwarded from your virtual Skype number to the Skype program on your computer.

18. Set your Skype program so it can send SMS messages directly from your computer. You can set it in such a way that the messages will seem to be coming from your cell-phone number. It is actually very convenient because you can type faster on the

computer's keyboard and you can send the same message to several people at once.

19. Do not carry the cell phone close to your body (e.g. in your pocket or on your belt). If you must carry it close to your body turn it off or switch it to air-plane mode. Use a radiation blocking case for carrying your mobile phone when it is not being used.

20. For some phone models you may be able to get a special radiation redirecting case compatible with your cell-phone model. These cases do not work by blocking the radiation but rather by redirecting it. They have a special purpose antenna built into the case structure that helps in diverting some of the radiation away from you. It also improves the cell-phone's reception and in this way allows the cell phone to transmit using lower radiation levels. The cell phone radiation redirecting cases are designed for specific cell phone makes and models. Accordingly, their effectiveness may vary. Some boast impressive radiation reduction for some phone models. However, you need to remember that lab tests have been made under ideal conditions. Real life conditions may reduce the effectiveness, especially if your body happens to be between your cell phone and the cell phone tower.

21. Do not stand or sit next to another person when he/she is using a cell phone. You may be exposed passively to radiation coming out of their phone (just like passive smoking). Don't get me wrong - I am not suggesting you get into a fight over this. Just get up and stand or sit somewhere else.

22. You also need to realize that if you are in a crowded public place with a lot of people around you - most of them probably have a cell phone in their pocket or bag. All these cell phones keep emitting short but powerful electromagnetic pulses in order to communicate with the closest cell phone tower. Radiation exposure is cumulative so the total radiation exposure resulting from these cell phones may be significant.

23. When travelling on a train or bus, the passengers' cell phones transmit electromagnetic pulses more frequently to establish connection with different cell phone towers as the bus or train moves quickly from one location to another. This may result in a dramatic increase in the total levels of EMR transmitted by the cell phones even if no one seems to be talking. In other words - on a crowded fast moving train or bus, you are exposed to a constant barrage of short sharp and powerful bursts of EMR. Public transport is for everyone, including babies, children, pregnant women, electro-sensitive people and immune compromised individuals. Laws should be put in place to require anyone carrying a cell phone to switch it to air-plane mode or turn it off - when boarding a bus or train.

High or low SAR – does it really matter?

SAR stands for "Specific Absorption Rate". This number is a measure of the rate at which electromagnetic radiation is absorbed by our body tissues when we are exposed to radio frequency (RF) electromagnetic radiation. Theoretically using a phone with a lower SAR implies a lower EMR exposure per time unit. However, the SAR number represents lab test results performed under ideal conditions. In reality various factors may change the picture dramatically and a lower SAR phone could sometimes emit more radiation than a higher SAR phone. How is this possible? Well – let's take a simple example: Some Smartphones have a very sophisticated adaptive transmission power control that monitors and modifies the transmitted radiation level according to reception conditions. If reception is very good (maximum number of bars on the reception display) it automatically reduces transmission power level to minimum. On the other hand, if reception is very poor, the phone will adapt accordingly and use a much higher transmission power (up to a 1000 times higher than the minimum level !!!). Older more "primitive" phones may not have adaptive transmission power technology built in and consequently they may always transmit at the maximum radiation level. As explained in detail in a previous section, the way you use the phone (e.g. SMS, using speakerphone, using an air-tube headset etc.) can have a huge impact on your radiation exposure, and is by far more significant than the phone's SAR rating. A technology naive person may take a low SAR number as an all clear sign and consequently end up with very high cumulative electromagnetic radiation (EMR) exposure.

What about Bluetooth headsets?

Bluetooth is a name given to wireless technology used for transmitting and receiving data over short distances. The radio frequency band used by Bluetooth devices is 2400–2480 MHz, quite similar to those used in some mobile phones. EMR levels emitted by Bluetooth devices are much lower than those emitted by mobile phones. Maximum power output from a Bluetooth class 1 device is 100 mW; from a class 2 device - 2.5 mW; and class 3 device 1 mW. However, as mentioned in previous sections radiation exposure depends not only on the power of the RF source but also on the distance between the body and the transmitting source. Bluetooth headsets work by transmitting and receiving RF to and from cell-phones and are usually positioned directly over the ear terminating inside the ear. Because of the close proximity to your head the Bluetooth headset exposes your brain to high levels of radiation.

Image 8.2 - Cell Phone RF radiation (measured during initial connection phase)Figure 8.1 Cell Phone

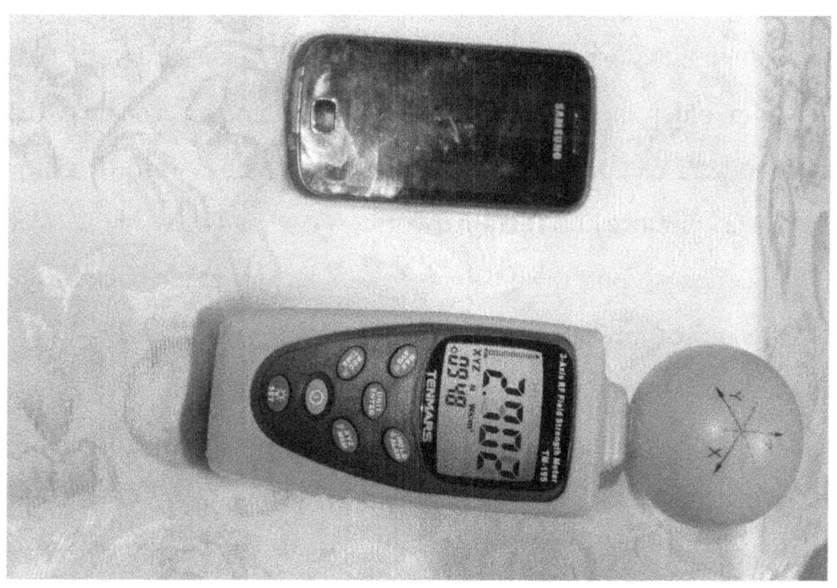

Figure 8.1 Radiation Protection Strategy

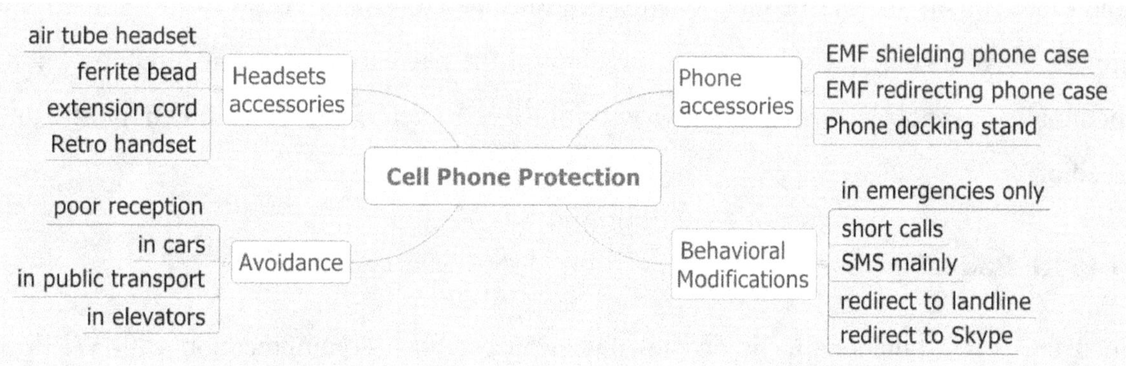

9 WI-FI EMF PROTECTION

What is Wi-Fi?

An important aspect of your EMF protection strategy is elimination of unnecessary sources of EMR within your living space or workspace. Most people are connected to the Internet via fiber optic cable or copper DSL (digital subscriber line) connected to a combination broadband modem and router. The router allows several computers to share a single Internet connection. In some cases, especially with older models, the router and modem are separate devices. Most recent routers and router-modems can be connected to computers using two different modes – wired local area network (LAN) or wireless local area network (WLAN). The wired network method relies on Ethernet cables that connect a port (also called jack or socket) at the back of the router to a similar port at the back (or side) of the laptop or desktop computer using an RJ-45 type connector. Most routers have four of these ports at the back (often in yellow color). The wireless connection between the router and computers is called a Wi-Fi connection (pronounced why fy and also spelled WiFi or Wifi). It uses RF (radio frequencies) in the microwave band similar to mobile phones, DECT phones and mobile base station towers. Wi-Fi usually uses the 2.4 GHz band but sometimes has a dual-band (2.4 GHz and 5 GHz). The Wi-Fi function can usually be turned on and off using a push button. A led light in the front of the unit will indicate that the Wi-Fi is on. In some older routers the Wi-Fi functionality can only be controlled via software. Some routers are wireless only, in other words they do not have Ethernet cable ports and obviously the Wi-Fi functionality cannot be turned off. Try to avoid any router if its Wi-Fi functionality cannot be turned off.

Wi-Fi RF Radiation

When the Wi-Fi functionality is on the router can establish communication with Wi-Fi enabled devices in range. If any of these devices requests to connect to the Internet, it is served by the router that transmits the information in chunks called data packets. The more data required, the more data packets need to be transmitted (e.g. - when downloading large files or viewing a video). If a computer is far away or blocked by obstacles (like walls), both computer and router increase RF transmission power output to overcome obstacles that may interfere with the communication. When sitting in close proximity to a wireless router with the Wi-Fi function enabled you may be exposed to a substantial amount of microwave radiation, comparable to exposure levels you may experience in close proximity to a cell phone tower.

Wi-Fi Radiation Protection Strategy

Many people have a wireless router in their office located next to their PC. The PC should be connected to the router using an Ethernet cable as explained above. However, the Wi-Fi function is often turned on regardless. This is unfortunate because often people mostly use one computer in the office and connect via mobile devices less frequently so they don't really need to be exposed to Wi-Fi RF radiation most of the time.

If members of your family are using computers in other rooms, the router will work harder (i.e. transmit higher levels of radiation) in order to overcome obstacles, provide a strong enough signal and communicate effectively with computers located in other rooms. The result is that anybody sitting next to the router is exposed to a high level of EMR.

Most people are not even aware of the fact that the Wi-Fi can be turned off by a simple push of a button. In some older routers there is no on-off button. In such cases turning the Wi-Fi off has to be done using your Internet browser to communicate with your router from your PC. For every router brand this may be done a little bit differently.

Here are the steps you need to take to minimize your Wi-Fi radiation exposure:

1. Connect your PC to your router using an Ethernet cable.

2. If you or family members use computers in other rooms to connect to the Internet frequently you need to run Ethernet cables from the router to other rooms. You can run them along the walls neatly concealed in aesthetic inexpensive plastic ducts. This will allow you to use the router with the Wi-Fi functionality turned off.

3. Refer to the user's manual and make sure you know what you are doing.

4. Back up your router settings before attempting to implement any changes because if you lose your settings you may not be able to reconnect to the Internet, and you will then need to call your Internet service provider's technical support and get assistance re-establishing the correct parameters on your modem-router. However, if you carefully back up your modem-router settings to a file saved on your computer, you will be able to reload the settings to your router from the backup file, reboot the router and recover the original settings.

5. Each router is different so you need to follow the manufacturer's instructions in your router's user manual. With my old router for example I type the URL **http://192.168.1.1/**. A little dialogue box pops up and asks me to provide **username** and **password**. After entering the correct username and password the router's control panel appears. I then click on the wireless tab and tick off the "Enable Wireless Router" box. I then need to restart my router. Hopefully, your router is newer and the Wi-Fi can be turned off with a simple push of a button.

6. To reduce your radiation exposure, you are advised to turn the Wi-Fi off as often as possible, especially when you are sitting right next to the router. Only **turn** on the Wi-Fi if you need to use a computer, tablet, Smartphone or other mobile devices in another room. Repeated RF measurements will allow you to identify EMF hotspots in your house and reduce exposure by repositioning your Wi-Fi router, computers and other equipment.

7. Some routers will enable the Wi-Fi functionality whenever they are turned off and on again, after being rebooted or after downloading a software or firmware update. Routers are often set to download these updates automatically and very frequently. The way to check if the Wi-Fi is on or off is to look at the router's front panel. The WLAN led should be off. If for some reason it is on, turn the Wi-Fi off again. This can be quite annoying because you often turn off the Wi-Fi only to discover an hour later that it has turned itself off again. The best solution for this is to get a router that does not have Wi-Fi functionality at all or at least a router that does not re-enable its Wi-Fi automatically.

Image 9.1 - Measuring Wi-Fi RF Radiation

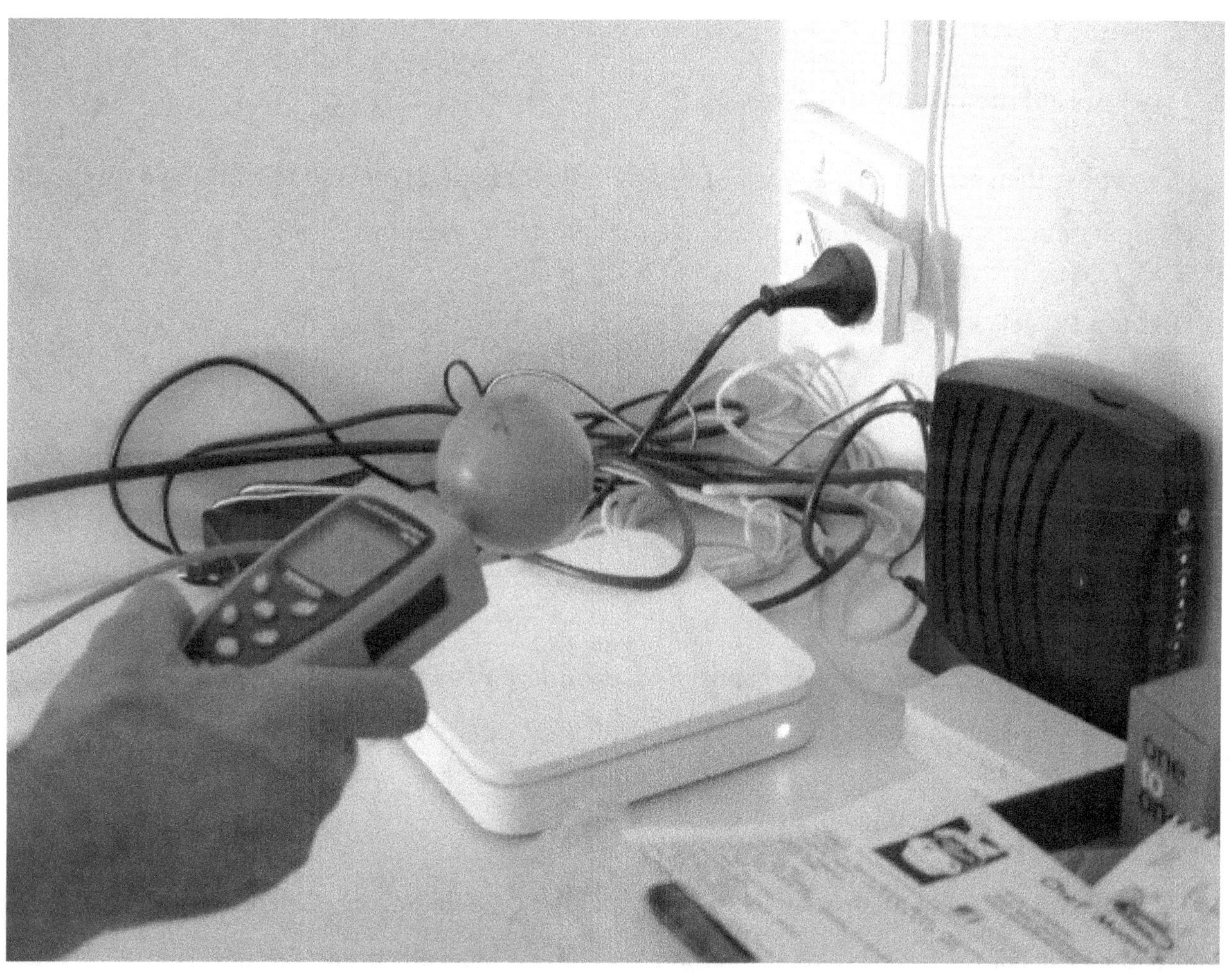

10 PC EMF PROTECTION

Types of radiation emitted by Desktop PCs

PCs expose the user to various types of EMF/EMR. Radiation type and level depend on the PC's configuration and use and each requires specific protection measures.

Desktop PC RF Radiation

Many PCs are Wi-Fi enabled. What this means is that they are able to connect to a wireless local area network (WLAN) by transmitting and receiving radio frequencies (RF). At the time of writing this article the most common WLAN frequency band in use is the 2.4 GHz band (i.e. 2.4 billion cycles per second). This frequency band is part of the microwave sector of the electromagnetic spectrum. Other microwave frequency bands that are often used for WLAN networks are 3.6 GHz, 4.9 GHz, and 5 GHz microwave bands. The good news is PCs' RF radiation can be eliminated completely in some cases and in other cases reduced as described later in this section.

Desktop PC LF Radiation

PCs contain a range of internal and external components including an AC adapter, a screen, fans, a processor, a hard drive, speakers, microphone, camera and electronic circuitry. Low frequency (LF) radiation is a by-product of the alternating electric (AC) current that flows into the PC (frequency is usually 50 or 60 Hz depending on the country you live in) and various direct currents (DC) flowing inside the PC. These currents create low frequency (LF) electromagnetic fields that are radiated from the PC causing increase in electromagnetic radiation exposure. The good news is that LF radiation diminishes rapidly as you increase your distance from the source. I will discuss this in detail below.

Desktop PCs cause dirty electricity

PCs internal electronic components also generate high frequency transients that often infiltrate your home's electrical network in the form of "dirty electricity". The good news is that your home can be protected effectively from dirty electricity coming from your PC as explained below.

PC Radiation Protection Strategies

PC RF radiation protection

Problem: The PC's Wi-Fi is enabled and you are being exposed to very significant levels of RF electromagnetic radiation.

Solutions:

1. If you are using your PC to connect to the Internet, then get a standard Ethernet cable (also called CAT 5e RJ45) and connect your PC directly to the router. Some Apple MAC computers may require a special adaptor to connect to a standard Ethernet cable. Consult your Apple dealer.

2. Turn off the Wi-Fi functionality of the PC. Each PC is different, but in general if you type the search keyword "wireless", you will probably be able to click on a program that controls the wireless function in your PC and turn it off. Consult the user's manual if you cannot find it.

3. Turn off the Wi-Fi functionality of the router. Some routers have a special button that enables turning the Wi-Fi off. Others may require turning the Wi-Fi off via the router's administration software installed on your computer. Please refer to the section explaining how to turn OFF the router's Wi-Fi functionality. Consult the user's manual if you cannot find it. Make sure the router's Wi-Fi functionality stays off as explained in the previous section.

4. You may also like to double check RF radiation levels around the router using an RF meter just to make sure the router is actually turned off. Similarly, check RF radiation levels

around the PC using the same RF meter.

5. Some routers can transmit on two different RF frequency bands. At times one band may be turned on and the other band turned off. To make extra sure both frequency bands are disabled you need to measure radiation levels using a wide range RF meter.

6. Get an RF EMF meter that can measure electromagnetic frequencies of up to 5.5 GHz at least. Many RF EMF meters can only detect and measure frequencies up to 3 or 3.3 GHz (this is enough to detect most Wi-Fi routers and cell phones but not for all Wi-Fi frequency bands).

PC LF Radiation Protection

PCs emit significant levels of low frequency (LF) radiation. There are several sources of LF radiation associated with PCs. These include the AC Adapter/power supply, the screen, the fans, and circuitry. Unlike RF radiation most sources of LF radiation cannot be turned off. However, there are steps that you can take to significantly reduce your level of LF electromagnetic radiation exposure. Each of these requires specific attention and protection. Taking the following measures will help you reduce your exposure to LF radiation emitted by the PC.

1. PCs are NOT usually connected to the electric socket via an external AC adapter that looks like a little black box (or little white box in some MAC Apple laptops and notebooks) as in most desktop computers the adapter is internal. However, whether located externally or internally these adapters may emit significant LF radiation. If they are old and/or slightly defective they may emit very high LF radiation.

2. The internal components of the PC emit LF electromagnetic radiation. Take the following steps to protect yourself

3. Always use a **wired** (NOT wireless!!!) mouse and keyboard equipped with sufficiently long cables. Position them on the desk. Position the PC as far from you on the desk as the cables allow.

4. If radiation levels around your body are still higher than ambient levels, you may use

the following additional measure:

5. Get a universal earthing mat. Connect it following manufacturer's instructions. Position the keyboard and mouse on top of the earthing mat. Re-test radiation levels. Whether or not this helps depends on your PC's configuration.

6. The PC and/or peripherals may be inducing an AC voltage in your body. Take the following steps to protect yourself:

7. Get an earthing mat. Connect it according to manufacturer's instructions.

8. Position the mat on the floor under your feet. Take off your shoes and socks and have your bare feet firmly on the mat. Earthing will reduce levels of AC voltage on your body.

9. The PC's electronic components may be generating high frequency transients that create dirty electricity in your home's electrical network. Take the following steps to protect yourself:

10. Get an extension cord with a multi-socket and plug it into the AC socket you intend to use for the PC.

11. Get a dirty electricity meter. Measure dirty electricity level in GS - Graham Stetzer units. It should be lower than 50 GS units.

12. Plug the PC into the multi-socket and remeasure using a dirty electricity meter. A significantly higher reading than before indicates the PC is polluting your electrical network with dirty electricity.

13. Get a dirty electricity filter and plug it into the socket. Re-measure dirty electricity level in GS (Graham Stetzer units) or similar measure. It should now be lower than 50 GS units.

11 LAPTOP EMF PROTECTION

Laptops and notebooks have become powerful enough to satisfy the computing needs of most people. They have also become affordable and consequently gained much popularity especially with the younger generation. The problem with laptops is that they expose the user to significant levels of electromagnetic radiation. Their compact structure and light weight may lead to a false belief that they are relatively EMF safe. However, using a laptop actually exposes you to higher levels of electromagnetic radiation (EMR) than using a bulkier desktop computer. There are several reasons for this and it is important to get a good grasp of the concepts as this will help you apply an effective laptop EMR defensive strategy and use your laptop safely. Laptops emit several types of EMR each requiring specific protection measures described next.

Laptop RF Radiation

Most if not all laptops are Wi-Fi enabled. What this means is that they are able to connect to a wireless local area network (WLAN) by transmitting and receiving radio frequencies (RF). At the time of writing this article the most common **WLAN frequency band in use is the 2.4 GHz** band (i.e. 2.4 billion cycles per second). This frequency band is part of the microwave sector of the electromagnetic spectrum. Other microwave frequency bands that are often used for WLAN networks are **3.6 GHz, 4.9 GHz, and 5 GHz microwave bands.** The good news is that laptops' RF radiation can be eliminated completely in some cases and in other cases reduced as described later in this section.

Laptop LF Radiation

Laptops contain a range of internal and external components including an AC adapter, a screen, fans, a processor, a hard drive, speakers, microphone, camera and electronic circuitry. Low frequency (LF) radiation is a by-product of the alternating electric (AC) current that flows into the laptop (frequency is usually **50 or 60 Hz** depending on the country you live in) and various direct currents (DC) flowing inside the laptop. These currents create low frequency (LF) electromagnetic fields that radiate from the laptop causing increased electromagnetic radiation exposure. The good news is that LF radiation diminishes rapidly as you increase your distance yourself from the source. I will discuss this in detail below.

Laptops cause dirty electricity

Laptops' internal electronic components also generate high frequency transients that often infiltrate your home's electrical network in the form of "dirty electricity". The good news is that your home can be protected effectively from dirty electricity generated by your laptop as explained below. Laptop Radiation Protection Strategies are described next.

Laptop RF radiation protection

Problem: The laptop's Wi-Fi is enabled and you are being exposed to very significant levels of RF electromagnetic radiation.

Solutions:

1. If you are using your laptop to connect to the Internet get a standard Ethernet cable (also called CAT 5e RJ45) and connect your laptop directly to the router. Some Apple MAC laptops may require a special adapter to connect the laptop to the standard Ethernet cable. Consult your Apple dealer.

2. Turn off the Wi-Fi functionality of the laptop. Each laptop is different. Some actually have a button above or below the keyboard for turning the Wi-Fi on and off. In general, if you type the search keyword "wireless", you will probably be able to click on a program that controls the wireless function in your laptop and turn it off. Consult the user's manual if you cannot find it

3. Turn off the Wi-Fi functionality of the router. Some routers have a special button that enables turning the Wi-Fi off. Others may require turning the Wi-Fi off via the router's administration software installed on your computer. Please refer to the section explaining how to turn OFF the router's Wi-Fi functionality. Consult the user's manual if you cannot find it.

4. Make sure the router's Wi-Fi functionality stays off as explained in the previous section.

5. You may also like to double check RF radiation levels around the router using an RF meter just to make sure the router is actually turned off. Similarly, check RF radiation levels around the laptop using the same RF meter.

6. Some routers can transmit on two different RF frequency bands. At times one band may be turned on and the other band turned off. To make extra sure both frequency bands are disabled you need to measure radiation levels using a wide range RF meter.

7. Get an RF EMF meter that can measure electromagnetic frequencies of up to 5.5 GHz at least. Many RF EMF meters can only detect and measure frequencies up to 3 or 3.3 GHz (this is enough to detect most Wi-Fi routers and cell phones but not for all Wi-Fi frequency bands).

8. If you are planning a trip you need to prepare in advance so you can connect to the Internet safely while away. Please read the section on EMF safe travel.

9. I suggest you always put your laptop on a desk and **not on your lap**. However, if you are on the road and this is the only way for your to use your laptop you can get a laptop anti-radiation pad that will at least shield your reproductive organs from direct exposure to the laptop. and will reduce some of the potential harm to your reproductive organs and to your future offspring However, you must realize that the rest of your body will still be exposed to EMR as it radiates in all directions. As mentioned above the further you are from the source of the radiation the lower your exposure so if your laptop is sitting on your lap your reproductive organs suffer the higher levels of radiation exposure.

10. If you are travelling or in a public library or coffee shop and have no other alternative but to connect your laptop to the WLAN via Wi-Fi, make sure the reception is good. You can tell by the number of bars on the Wi-Fi icon on the screen. Do not connect if the reception is poor as in some cases this may result in higher radiation levels being emitted from the laptop's Wi-Fi.

Laptop LF Radiation Protection

Laptops emit significant levels of low frequency (LF) radiation. There are several sources of LF radiation associated with laptops. These include the laptops AC Adapter/power supply, the screen, the fans, and circuitry. Unlike RF radiation most sources of LF radiation in the laptop cannot be turned off. However, there are steps that you can take to significantly reduce your level of LF electromagnetic radiation exposure. Each of these requires specific attention and protection. Taking the following measures will help you reduce your exposure to LF radiation emitted by the laptop.

External AC adapters

Most laptops are connected to the electric socket via an external AC adapter that usually looks like a little black box (or little white box in some MAC Apple laptops and notebooks). These adapters may emit significant LF radiation. If they are old and/or slightly defective they may emit very high LF radiation. Take the following steps to protect yourself

1. Measure LF radiation levels close to the AC adapter using an LF EMF meter. The magnetic field directly next to the adapter should not exceed 2-3 Milligauss. If it exceeds 3 Milligauss you may consider testing similar adapters and perhaps getting a new adapter.

2. Move the AC adapter as far away from you as possible. It usually comes with a long cord that will allow positioning it at least one meter away. Then retest LF radiation levels close to your body to make sure they have dropped considerably. Hopefully readings close to your body will be similar to the general ambient levels of magnetic EMR in the room.

The internal components of the laptop emit LF electromagnetic radiation.

Your hands are positioned directly on top of the keyboard and exposed to high levels of LF radiation. Radiation exposure may affect the nerves and the blood supply running through your fingers. Since the blood circulates throughout the body, exposing the fingers to EMR will eventually affect every blood cell in your body. Take the following steps to protect yourself.

1. Measure radiation levels using an LF EMF meter. Disconnect the laptop from the AC power supply and use it on battery power. This may reduce levels of LF EMR.

2. Measure radiation levels again using an LF EMF meter. Radiation may still be too high. In that case, purchase a wired (NOT wireless!!!) mouse, keyboard and perhaps also an external LCD display. The external display, mouse and keyboard should be equipped with sufficiently long cables. Connect the keyboard, mouse and external display to the laptop. Position them in front of you on the desk. Position the laptop as far from you on the desk as the cables allow. Position the AC adapter as far from you as its cable allows. Re-test radiation levels. Hopefully readings will be much lower and similar to the general ambient level of EMR in the room.

Some laptops are not grounded.

In other words, the power cord connecting the laptop to the AC adapter only has two pins and two wires and not three pins and three wires as in grounded laptops. Laptops that are not grounded emit higher levels of EMR than grounded laptops. Take the following steps to protect yourself.

1. Apply the same procedure described above. In other words, test radiation levels, connect the laptop to an external wired keyboard, mouse and LCD display and position the laptop as far away from you as the keyboard and external display screen cords allow.

2. If radiation levels around your body are still higher than ambient levels, you may use the following additional measure. Get a universal earthing mat. Connect it following manufacturer's instructions. Position the laptop on top of the earthing mat. Re-test radiation levels. Whether or not this helps depends on your laptop's configuration. This is only an additional measure and not a substitute for using an external keyboard, mouse and display.

The laptop and/or peripherals may be inducing an AC voltage in your body.

Take the following steps to protect yourself:

1. Get a universal earthing mat. Connect it according to manufacturer's instructions.

2. Position the mat on the floor under your feet. Take off your shoes and socks and have your bare feet firmly on the mat. Earthing will reduce levels of AC voltage on your body.

The laptop's electronic components may be generating high frequency transients that create dirty electricity in your home's electrical network.

Take the following steps to protect yourself:

1. Get an extension cord with a multi-socket and plug it into the AC socket you intend to use for the laptop.

2. Get a dirty electricity meter. Measure dirty electricity level in GS (Graham Stetzer) units. Reading should be below 50 GS units.

3. Plug the laptop into the multi-socket and remeasure using the dirty electricity meter. A significantly higher reading than before indicates the laptop is polluting your electrical network with dirty electricity.

4. Get a dirty electricity filter and plug it into the socket. Re-measure dirty electricity level in GS units. It should now be below 50 GS units.

12 TABLET EMF PROTECTION

Tablets as the name implies are compact tablet shaped computers that are very portable and may be operated while holding the tablet with both hands close to the body. Tablets were created to fill the gap between laptops and Smartphones. As such tablets share many of the characteristics of both laptops and Smartphones and also emit the same types of electromagnetic radiation. Most tablets emit two types of electromagnetic radiation that we need to protect against. These are radio frequency (RF) radiation and low frequency (LF) electromagnetic radiation. The purpose of this section is to help you reduce your electromagnetic radiation exposure when using tablet computers.

Tablet electromagnetic radiation

Most tablets are only intended to be used as Wi-Fi enabled devices. Some of the more expensive tablets are capable of operating both as a Wi-Fi enabled device and as a Smartphone. If you are using your tablet with a cell-phone SIM card, you may refer to the section on cell-phone radiation protection. Typically, though tablets are used to connect to the Internet via a Wi-Fi network (WLAN) at home, at the office, in coffee shops and other public places. Wi-Fi connection requires the tablet to transmit and receive radio frequencies (RF) in the Wi-Fi RF band in most cases these Wi-Fi networks operate on the 2.4 GHz (2.4 Billion cycles per second) band but in some cases may also operate on higher bands.

Radiation exposure when using a tablet

Tablets' compact and sleek design may be misleading as we are exposed to substantial levels of EMR when using them. Similar levels of RF radiation are emitted by both tablets and laptops. LF radiation levels emitted by tablets are lower than those emitted by laptops because tablets are smaller and therefore consume less power. Tablets are normally used on battery mode whereas laptops are often used while plugged into the electric socket. However, the big difference between tablets and laptops is the way we use them. Tablets are often used while holding them with both hands and because they have smaller screens people often hold them quite close to the head to see better. As explained in previous sections if you half your distance from the tablet to your head you quadruple your radiation exposure and this is exactly the problem with using tablets.

Tablet Radiation Protection Strategy

You can reduce your EMR exposure when using a tablet by taking the following steps:

1. When at home or at the office - turn the tablet off and connect to the internet using a computer.

2. If you want to watch videos on your tablet, do not download them to the tablet via a Wi-Fi connection. First, download the video from the internet to your computer with the router connected to the PC using an Ethernet cable connection and the router's Wi-Fi turned off. Next, transfer the downloaded files from your computer to the tablet using a USB cable. This will enable you to download large files while avoiding exposure to significant levels of Wi-Fi RF radiation.

3. When watching a video on the tablet, do not hold it in your hands. Position the tablet on a special stand so you don't have to hold it all the time. This will also ease the stress and strain to your arms, shoulders and neck. Some tablet cases have a built in folding stand that allows using the tablet hands free. Some of these cases also improve cellular signal, Wi-Fi reception and range, while reducing exposure to potentially harmful radiation.

4. If you must put the tablet on your lap, it is highly recommended that you get a radiation protection shield or pad. Position the pad between the tablet and your lap. This will protect your reproductive organs from radiation exposure and reduce the risk of cancer and infertility. However, you need to realize that the rest of your body will still be exposed to electromagnetic radiation.

5. If you are pregnant don't use a tablet. Please refer to the section on Pre and Post Natal EMF protection for more details.

NOTE: As tablets are similar to laptops in many ways and you can find more information on protection strategies in the section dealing with laptop radiation protection.

13 SMART METERS EMF PROTECTION

What are "smart" meters?

Installation of so-called "smart meters" by the utility companies has been gaining much publicity in recent years. Smart meters are only one of several serious electromagnetic radiation hazards in our lives. However, in most cases they are being forced on consumers and perhaps this explains why so many people are getting organized and trying to opt out. For the benefit of those who are not familiar with smart meters let's just define smart meters as utility meters (electricity, water and gas) that have a two-way communication with a central system to enable frequent and accurate collection of data on usage levels and patterns. There are many problems with these meters including health concerns, privacy concerns and increased cost to the consumer.

Smart meters emit pulsed wireless RF radiation

The main concern with so-called "smart" meters is that they communicate using pulsed wireless RF (radio frequency) technology that many scientists believe to be a serious health risk factor. Furthermore, many individuals around the world are already reporting serious adverse health events associated with the installation of smart meters on their property. Some have reported having to move out of their homes in an attempt to regain their health.

Smart meters may also generate dirty electricity

Smart meters may contaminate your home network with dirty electricity in two ways:

1. Smart meters emit frequent bursts of pulsed RF electromagnetic radiation. Because the smart meter is connected to your home electrical network, the electrical wiring throughout the house becomes an antenna that receives bursts of pulsed RF, carries them to every part of your home and then radiates the energy as EMF throughout your home.

2. Smart meters are computerized electronic devices with electronic circuits that are coupled to

your electrical network. If they do not incorporate special filters this may result in high frequency micro-surges superimposing themselves on the "normal" AC electricity in your network creating "dirty electricity".

Prevention is better than cure

Prevention is always preferable to cure. This is also the case with smart meters. It is important to try to take proactive preventive measures in a timely fashion. There are various avenues of action, including contacting your elected representatives, contacting various citizen rights organizations, joining local groups and alerting the media.

If you are electro-hypersensitive, or suffer from another health condition, you may be able to get a written report from a medical specialist specifying why the installation of a smart meter may cause significant deterioration in your existing medical condition(s). You need to keep a daily log of your symptoms and other details of your medical condition prior to the installation of the smart meter and to continue logging the details daily thereafter. You should also purchase a reasonable quality RF meter and record RF (radio frequency) EMF radiation levels prior to installation of the smart meter and then continue recording EMF levels thereafter. These records in conjunction with expert medical reports and other supporting material may serve as evidence in case you have no alternative but to take legal action.

The success of the aforementioned steps depends on many factors, including the legal situation in your state or country, the level of support you will be able to get and your individual situation. Even if you intend to take legal action you still need to keep harmful electromagnetic radiation away from you while you are engaged in the process because there is no telling how long it will take and what the outcome might be. Therefore, it is essential to have a good complementary action plan. It is important to have a plan that is both radiation effective and cost-effective (i.e. not too expensive).

Smart Meter Protection Action Plan

The Smart meter protection action plan consists of two phases- a data gathering phase and a radiation protection phase.

Phase A - Data gathering

1. Get a reasonable quality RF meter (it doesn't have to be professional grade)

2. Take accurate measurements of maximum and average RF radiation levels inside your house and outside your house in all rooms but in particular inside and outside the wall where the utility company is proposing to install the smart meter. Since smart meters transmit short bursts of pulses every X number of minutes, your RF meter needs to be able to record continuously over a time frame of at least $10X$ minutes. For example, if the smart meter transmits every 2 minutes, you need to record over a period of 20 minutes at least. Ideally, you should be able to record continuously over a 24-hour period, but that may require using a professional grade meter mostly used by EMF consultants. You need to take these measurements several times during the day and night. For example, in the early morning, mid-morning, noon, midafternoon, evening, night, and midnight. I suggest you use a spreadsheet (a big table with rows and columns) to record your measurement results. You can use Microsoft® Excel® or the Free Open Office® Calc® Spreadsheet. Alternately you can get a free Google® account and log in, click on Google **Drive**, then click on **Create**, and select **Spreadsheet**. A new spreadsheet will be created and then you can start recording the data.

3. Allocate a row for each measurement time, (e.g. 6 AM, 9 AM, 12 Noon, 3 PM, 6 PM, 9 PM, 12 Midnight). Allocate columns for measurement locations (e.g. bedroom 1, bedroom 2, bedroom 3, living room, dining room, kitchen, bathroom 1, bathroom 2, garage, back yard, front yard etc.). In each location first measure in the center of the room, then next to a window, above the beds, desks and other locations where people spend much time. Please note if there are significant differences within rooms and between rooms.

4. After the smart meter has been installed continue taking accurate measurements of EMR levels inside your house and outside your house in all rooms and log them as described above.

Phase B - Radiation protection

Assuming your measurements have shown an increase in EMR levels after the smart meter has been installed you need to take protective measures. The following action plan has several steps. After executing each step, you need to re-measure radiation levels. If radiation levels are back to what they were before the smart meter was installed, you can suspend further action and adopt and wait and measure approach. If the EMR levels are still higher than before, you may proceed to the next step. Taking this approach may help you save unnecessary expenses and work.

1. Significant electromagnetic radiation may enter the house via the windows. If the smart meter is attached to a wall that has a window, you may consider installing a window mosquito net/mesh that is made of metallic material NOT plastic. Measure the radiation levels before installing the insect mesh and then measure the radiation levels in the room after installing it. The metallic mesh has RF radiation blocking properties. Depending on the location of the meter in relation to the window this may or may not be sufficient to secure your window from EMF radiation.

2. If radiation still enters the room via the window, you may consider purchasing an RF radiation blocking fabric and using it to make a curtain for that window. Make the curtain wider and taller than the dimensions of the window to prevent EMR leakage between the curtain and the window frame. This additional curtain will significantly reduce any residual EMF still entering via the window.

3. Now measure residual EMF radiation levels in the room again. The amount of radiation entering via the wall depends very much on the material the wall is made of. Heavy concrete walls may block 90% of the radiation or more. Walls made of lighter materials may behave as a transparent material (i.e. the radiation will go through them unimpeded). If levels of radiation in the room are still not back to normal you need to paint the wall inside the house with RF radiation shielding paint. Before you start However, please read the section that discusses how to apply RF shielding paint.

4. There are various types of EMF shielding paints. The better ones can also shield against low level LF (low frequency) radiation formed around electrical wires. Look for an RF

shielding paint that is a pure acrylic (i.e. not oil based) paint, can be used both indoors and outdoors, has good humidity resistance and good tensile strength and durability. Most RF paints come in 1 liter and 5 liter containers. A one-liter container will usually provide one coat for an area of 7.5 square meters (indoors) and 5 square meters (outdoors). For example, a wall that is 2.5 meters in height and 3 meters in width has an area of 7.5 square meters (2.5 X 3 = 7.5). A 5-liter container will provide a single coat for an area of roughly 37.5 square meters or two coats for an area of almost 19 square meters. A single coat (layer) of a good RF shielding paint may provide an attenuation of 38 dB (i.e. shielding effectiveness of 99.984 %), and a double coat (two layers) may provide an attenuation of 45 dB (i.e. shielding effectiveness of 99.997 %). This means that if you paint the wall inside the house you will be able to block almost all of the smart meter's RF radiation. The better EMF blocking paints also provide some shielding against low frequency EMF created by the electrical wiring connected to the meter, although that is not the main cause of concern here.

BEFORE applying the RF shielding paint you need to have a certified electrician prepare the grounding for the paint as an RF shielding paint must always be grounded following manufacturer's instructions.

5. The next step is to apply one coat of RF shielding paint and let it dry. After it dries, measure the residual RF EMF radiation inside the room.

6. If the result is satisfactory you may then apply a top coating – preferably a plastic bonded water-based emulsion paint, facade paint or silicon resin paint. You probably need to apply at least 3 layers of top coating as RF shield paints are usually made black on purpose – to help you visually verify that you have covered the wall completely without leaving any gaps for the EMR to leak through.

7. If you wish to get an even greater level of attenuation you can apply a second coat of shielding paint **BEFORE** applying the top cover.

8. **NOTE: ONLY a certified electrician** should connect and test any grounding accessories. Electricity may cause electrocution, serious injuries or death. **Do not attempt to do any electrical work by yourself!**

14 BEDROOM EMF PROTECTION STRATEGY

The bedroom's most important function is to provide conditions for good restorative sleep. Sleep is essential to maintain and restore good health. During sleep the body recovers and repairs itself while the mind attempts to digest and reassess information absorbed during the waking state. Many psychological processes take place, some manifesting in forms of dreams. Presence of EMF/EMR in the bedroom may cause poor non-restorative sleep, sleep disturbances and even sleep disorders. Therefore, you need to make sure that your bedroom is EMF safe.

Devices such as smart meters, mobile devices and Wi-Fi routers emit short powerful pulses frequently when turned ON. Some scientists now believe that EMR, specifically short frequent powerful pulses of microwave radiation may affect the pineal gland in the brain in a similar way that light does. The presence of light delays the production of melatonin by the pineal gland. Melatonin is a master hormone and powerful antioxidant with many key physiological functions. Melatonin helps us fall asleep and stay asleep. It also has an important role in cancer prevention.

Follow these steps to make your bedroom EMF safe

1. Before going to bed turn off routers, cell phones, DECT phones and other devices or move them out of the room.

2. Do not use an electric alarm clock. Use a battery operated alarm clock and position it far away from you.

3. Make sure all the power sockets have on/off safety switches. Before going to bed make sure all sockets in the bedroom that have electrical devices plugged in are switched off. This will reduce residual EMF in the room as electrical devices tend to generate low EMF when plugged in even if they are not turned on.

   NOTE: This does not apply to emergency and medical devices that need to be ON all the time. For example, if you are using a CPAP machine to control sleep Apnoea, the device must be on and continue operating. Always follow your doctor's instructions.

4. If your AC power sockets do not have on/off safety switches you can connect electrical devices via power boards that have a safety on/off switch.

5. Install an on-demand switch next to your main power box. This switch will disconnect any branch of your electrical network that is not consuming any power. This will reduce residual EMF levels in your bedroom at night.

6. Choose the position of your bed carefully. Make sure it is far from sources of EMR such as power boxes, air-conditioning systems, heating systems, solar system inverters, refrigerators or Wi-Fi routers on the other side of the wall.

7. Neutralizing dirty electricity in the bedroom should be a priority. This can be done by installing dirty electricity filters. However, these filters may generate low levels of LF radiation so you need to position your bed at least 1 meter away from dirty electricity filters. Use an LF gauss meter to determine LF radiation safe zones.

8. Shielding the bedroom from RF should be a priority. Please refer to a previous section.

9. Measure RF radiation levels again. If RF radiation levels in the room are still too high, you may consider hanging an RF shielding canopy over your bed. The canopy will provide an RF safe sleeping space if no RF radiation is coming from below.

10. Measure RF radiation levels again. If RF radiation is also coming from below (for example if you are sleeping directly above a Wireless router installed in the apartment below you) you must also spread an RF shielding fabric or mat under the bed. Unless you do that, the canopy may actually increase your RF radiation exposure by reflecting RF radiation coming from below back at you

15 TEST BEFORE YOU BUY OR RENT

Initial Information gathering

When it comes to buying or renting property - location is a prime consideration. This is also true with regards to EMF safety. Choosing an EMF safe location should be a prime consideration because all EMF design and protection measures may not be adequate to counteract the effect of powerful EMF/EMR sources.

You should acquire as much information as you can with regards to plans to construct hi-tension power lines, cell phone towers, telecommunication towers, TV or radio stations and radar stations in that area. Each of these EMF hazards has a different safety radius that needs to be taken into consideration.

If you feel confident about your ability to measure EMF radiation (LF, RF and dirty electricity) conduct initial measurements and rule out properties that have pervasive high LF and/or RF radiation. You can also rule out properties that have a lot of EMF/EMR hotspots that would require substantial investment to fix.

Getting an EMF consultant to write a report for every property you consider buying or renting may be expensive. You can save money by narrowing down the options by eliminating properties that have obvious EMF problems. Rule out properties that are located in close proximity to obvious present or future EMF hazards such as cell-phone towers, hi-tension power lines and the like.

The next step after narrowing down your options is to get an EMF consultant to conduct thorough measurements and write a report on a property you are seriously considering buying or renting.

Pre-purchase or Pre-rent professional EMF Report

As discussed above, before buying land or a property it is highly recommended that you hire an EMF professional to conduct a thorough EMF survey outside and inside as well as in the surrounding neighborhood.

The report should include:

1. All types of electromagnetic radiation (LF, RF and dirty electricity)

2. Average maximum and minimum radiation levels over an adequate time period

3. Radiation hotspots in each of the rooms and yard

4. Radiation levels in comparison to average levels in similar properties and in comparison to recommended safety levels.

5. Possible EMF protection strategy and estimated EMR levels inside the house after taking recommended measures

6. Estimated costs of suggested EMF protection strategy

7. Present and future EMF hazards affecting the property

16 DESIGNING AN EMF SAFE HOME

Building Biology

If you are considering building a new home from the ground up, then you are in a great position to design and construct a healthy living and working space for yourself following the principles of Building Biology. This is a relatively new area and well beyond the scope of this book. It focuses on the affects buildings have on the health of occupants. In recent years, a growing number of architects and builders have been incorporating building biology principles into their work.

Building Biology has several focus areas including:

1. Creating an EMF safe living environment

2. Using healthy nontoxic building materials

3. Creating a well ventilated space with good air quality

4. Creating a low noise space

5. Creating a living environment that enhances relaxation and reduces stress

Examples of EMF safe building design considerations

1. These are just some examples of EMF safe building design consideration that you may apply when designing a new house. A building biology consultant will be able to tailor the right solution for your specific requirements and needs. It is not advisable to do it yourself unless you are also a professional in a related field.

2. Electric power cable entry points into the house should be as far as possible from sleep, living, or work areas.

3. Power boxes should be as far as possible from sleep, living, or work areas.

4. Air-conditioning systems electrical components (e.g. motors, compressors, fans) should be as far as possible from sleep, living, or work areas.

5. Heating systems electrical components (e.g. motors, heating elements, fans) should be as far as possible from sleep, living, or work areas.

6. Washing machines and dryers should be as far as possible from sleep, living, or work areas. Dryers should have an external vent.

7. Dishwashers and refrigerators should be positioned away from the dining area

8. Refrigerators should not be positioned on the other side of a wall next to sleep, living, or work areas

Using EMF safe building technologies, gadgets and materials

Here are some examples of EMF safe building technologies that may be used. A building biology consultant can tailor the right solution for your specific requirements and needs. It is not advisable to do it yourself unless you are also a professional in a related field.

1. The walls, ceilings and roof should have thermal insulation using materials with good RF shielding properties.

2. Use low EMF electrical wires.

3. Install Ethernet cables and connections throughout the house to connect all computers and other devices using a fully wired non-radiation network. Connect the network to a central ADSL or cable modem and router to allow connecting to the Internet from every room using the fully wired non-radiation network.

4. Install a central on-demand automatic switch next to the power box.

5. All sockets should have their own safety switch.

6. Install fly screens made from metallic meshes with good RF shielding properties.

7. Install curtains with good RF shielding properties.

8. Install windows coated with special film that has good RF shielding properties.

9. Install Dirty Electricity suppression filters throughout the house.

10. Use RF shielding paints to protect walls where necessary

17 EMF SAFE TRAVEL

Travel exposes us to substantial amounts of EMF radiation. Here are some steps you can take to reduce EMF exposure while travelling:

1. Don't forget to take with you an air-tube headset, cell phone radiation blocking case and headset extension cord.

2. Make sure you book a Wi-Fi free accommodation. Some old hotels and B&B may still be Wi-Fi free.

3. Travel with a small pack of thermal blankets made of aluminium foil. These are light and compact, inexpensive, and can keep you warm and shield against RF radiation.

4. Travel with a three-meter-long Ethernet extension cable. In some hotels, the Wi-Fi is transmitted from a Wi-Fi router positioned on the desk in your room. Try to find a button that allows turning the wireless function off and disable the Wi-Fi functionality. Use your long Ethernet cable to connect your laptop to one of the spare ports at the back of the router.

5. Mobile phones generate substantial amounts of microwave radio frequency (RF) radiation. Try to use landlines wherever possible. You can also use Skype or similar software from your laptop to reduce your usage of your mobile phone. Before going on your trip make sure your Skype account is set up to make phone calls and has enough credit in it.

6. Disconnect any bed side electric alarm clocks. All hotels have these and they generate constant low frequency (LF) radiation.

7. Try to sit at the back of the air-plane. There is usually less EMF radiation there.

8. Try to sit away from plane engines. These produce substantial EMF.

9. Try to sit away from the cockpit and front of the plane. The communication and radar equipment produce substantial EMF.

10. For longer trips take your EMF meters with you. These will help you choose optimal accommodation and positioning within hotel rooms.

11. Use EMF shielding hats and clothing

18 EMF PROTECTION IN CARS

Cars generate a range of electromagnetic fields that can be broadly classified as LF and RF fields. Most people cannot sense these electromagnetic fields and are therefore not aware of their presence. However, as with any type of EMF these fields may also result in adverse health effects especially for electro-hypersensitive people.

Hybrid cars have fuel engines and smaller electric motors. The latter generates considerable EMR. Electric cars have much larger electric motors than hybrid cars and therefore generate much stronger EMR. Radiation exposure varies considerably from car to car and also depends on the location inside the car. In fuel engine cars, people sitting in the front seats are exposed to higher levels of EMR with the driver usually being exposed to highest levels of EMR. However, in hybrid cars and in electric cars EMR exposure depends on the exact configuration and location of the electric motor(s) and battery.

LF radiation sources in cars

LF sources in cars include the electrical system and often the car's radial tires when the car is in motion. The car's electrical system includes various components including the battery, power cables, lights, alternator, distributor and ignition fuses. They all emit EMR. When the headlights are on the cables connected to the battery emit higher levels of EMR. Radiation exposure varies considerably from car to car and also depends on the location inside the car. The only way to verify radiation levels is to measure using an LF radiation meter. Hybrid cars produce higher LF radiation than fuel only cars. Electric cars produce even higher LF radiation.

It may come as a surprise to most drivers but radial tires might generate considerable magnetic fields. These fields are caused because the steel wires in the radial tires become magnetized with use. As the tire rotates the magnetized wires generate alternating magnetic fields that can have strength of up to 1mG. These magnetic fields are stronger close to the tires but can be detected throughout the car.

RF radiation sources in cars

RF sources in cars include cell phones, Wi-Fi, Bluetooth and a range of electronic gadgetry such as GPRS/GSM/GPS systems. Some Wi-Fi systems installed in cars are so powerful that they can be received 300 meters away from the car. Imagine the exposure levels inflicted on the passengers by such a system. Cars are essentially metallic boxes on wheels. The metallic structure traps much of RF radiation transmitted from all sources inside the car. The trapped radiation bounces from side to side and from roof to floor until it is absorbed or until it exits via the windows. This significantly increases the passengers' exposure to RF radiation.

Road safety systems

Road safety and accident prevention is of utmost importance as it can save lives and prevent serious injuries. Therefore, having such a system installed in your car is of great benefit. Comparing these systems is well beyond the scope of this book and new types are coming out all the time. However, it is worth pointing out that some systems are radar-based and others are camera-only optical systems. Each of these systems probably has advantages and disadvantages. Obviously the radar-based systems work by transmitting pulses of microwave RF radiation. Assessing radar radiation exposure may require a specialized professional grade RF meter.

Car radiation protection strategy

The following steps will contribute to a significant reduction of your EMR exposure while inside cars:

1. Only use your cell phone inside the car in an emergency.

2. If you can then set your cell-phone to air-plane mode when in the car.

3. Install a hands-free kit for your cell phone. Connect the hands-free kit to an external antenna. The antenna should ideally be installed on the car's rooftop. The hands-free kit and the external antenna should be connected via a wire and not via Bluetooth. These measures will redirect much of the cell-phone's radiation away from you. However, you should still try to minimize using your cell-phone when in the car for safety reasons.

4. Do not use Wi-Fi or Bluetooth devices in the car. If the car already has Wi-Fi and/or Bluetooth functionality, get your car electrician to disable them.

5. Before buying a car go for a test drive and measure RF and LF radiation levels. Get the salesperson to drive the car while you conduct the measurements.

6. Many new cars are loaded with electronic gadgetry. The question you need to ask yourself is: *Do I really need all these gadgets?* By opting out of optional gadgets that are not really useful you may save money and reduce EMF levels inside the car.

7. If you are thinking of buying an electric or a hybrid car, take it for a test drive. Have the salesperson drive the car while you measure radiation levels. Focus on LF radiation levels and compare the results to those you recorded in similar fuel-only cars. Hybrid cars and electric cars are "greener" and may contribute to reduction of air-pollution in urban areas. However, you need to make sure that your EMF/EMR exposure does not increase significantly as a result of using electric or hybrid vehicles.

19 EMF PROTECTION ON PUBLIC TRANSPORTATION

EMR sources on public transportation

1. The main RF sources on buses and trains are passengers' cell phones and Wi-Fi.

2. The main LF sources on buses and trains are wheels that incorporate metallic material, electric motors and electrical components.

3. The main RF sources on planes are Wi-Fi, telecommunication equipment and radars. Some airlines have been introducing Wi-Fi that can also be accessed by passengers with mobile devices.

4. The main LF sources on planes are engines, heating systems and air-conditioning systems.

EMF issues on public transport

Public transport includes buses, trains, planes and ships. These are all constructed of various metals that have RF reflective properties. Increasingly Wi-Fi is made available on many forms of public transport. Most travellers also carry their cell-phones with them and often use their Smartphones to connect to the Internet directly or via Wi-Fi. The metal structure of buses, trains and planes reflects much of the Wi-Fi and cell-phone radiation and causes it to bounce back and forth inside the cabin. This significantly increases the passengers' radiation exposure. Furthermore, the metallic structure often creates poor reception on buses and trains and that may result in cell phones ramping up radiation levels to overcome obstacles. This also contributes to a significant increase in EMR exposure. Furthermore, public transport involves spending time in a confined space with a large number of people; buses and trains move at relatively high speed and a result the passengers' cell-phones constantly transmit RF pulses to sync with the closest cell phone tower. This also contributes to an increase in EMR exposure.

RF protection strategy on public transport

1. The best strategy is avoidance. Put simply – try to minimize your use of public transport especially if you suffer from EHS.

2. Turn your phone off or use it on air-plane mode to avoid it pulsing constantly close to your body as explained above.

3. Try to sit as far away as you can from other passengers. If the passenger sitting next to you is using a cell phone find another place to sit

4. You can also wear EMF protective clothing when using buses or trains.

5. Someone asked me if EMF protective clothing might create a problem with airport screening machines. To be honest - I don't know and it may also depend on the type of fibers used in the clothing and the screening machine itself. However, the most simple solution is to take with you an EMF shielding poncho and several aluminum thermal blankets and put them in your hand luggage. You can wear the poncho and cover yourself with the thermal blanket once you have boarded.

6. **NOTE**: EMF shielding poncho and thermal blankets will keep you safe from RF radiation but are not effective against LF radiation or cosmic radiation. You still need to sit as far away as you can from LF radiation sources such as engines and motors.

7. Try to sit or stand as far away from trains' or buses' motors or engines

8. Try to sit or stand as far away from trains' or buses' wheels

9. Try to sit or stand as far away from trains' or buses' Wi-Fi routers

10. On airplanes sit far away from the engines, cockpit and galleys. These have various sources of RF radiation. The cockpit has communication and electronics equipment. The radar is often mounted somewhere in the fuselage in the front of the plane. The galleys have various sources of LF radiation including heating elements used for preparing the meals. The engines may also be generating substantial LF magnetic radiation.

20 EMF Protective Clothing

EMF protective clothing provides some measure of protection against RF radiation. The clothing is made from RF shielding fabrics. These fabrics are generally made of a fine mesh of metallic fibres (e.g. copper, silver) interwoven into cotton and/or synthetic materials. It is the copper or silver fibres that provide the RF reflecting quality that these fabrics possess.

Good quality EMF protective clothing may be expensive. Furthermore, since clothing needs to be washed on a regular basis you may require several sets. Frequent washing may degrade the RF protective properties of the fabrics. It is always wise to contact the manufacturer to find out how many times you can wash the clothing before it loses its RF protective qualities.

EMF/EMR awareness is growing and more products are appearing on the market all the time. There are several types of EMF protective clothing. At the time of writing this book the majority of the products on the market are intended to be used by pregnant women to provide protection to the fetus. Pre- and Post-natal protection is discussed in detail in a subsequent section.

If you are Electro Hypersensitive (EHS), then RF protective clothing may allow you to step out of your house more often. However, because RF radiation levels in the environment are growing constantly with the introduction of faster and more powerful mobile telecommunication technologies, you may find the clothing will not be able to provide the same level of protection in the future as they do now.

Here are the most useful types of RF protective clothing:

RF protective hats and caps

Caps and hats protect the head from EMF coming from above such as from nearby antennas. They are also good against the sun. Care should be taken never to use a cell-phone with these caps on because the cap will reflect the cell-phone's radiation back and effectively increase EMR density inside the skull. These caps and hats should also not be worn close to a low lying source of EMF such as a router positioned on the floor, or EMF coming from an apartment on the floor below.

RF protective ponchos

Ponchos are very effective and also cost effective because they cover most of the body including the head, are worn over other clothing so do not require frequent washing and can fit most body sizes.

RF protective jackets

Jackets are also very effective and cost effective because they cover most of the upper body, are worn over other clothing so do not require frequent washing.

RF protective shirts

Shirts protect the upper body. The problem with shirts is that they need to be changed and washed frequently. This means that you have to buy several and the total cost may be significant

RF protective pants

Pants protect the lower body. They may add protection to areas not covered by ponchos or jackets

RF protective dresses

Some EMF protective dresses cover most of the body. There is a range of maternity dresses available to protect both mother and fetus. This is discussed in detail in a subsequent section.

21 Pre & Post - natal EMF Protection

Pre- and post-natal EMF health risks

We are all exposed to a growing number of EMF sources in our daily lives. Radiation levels are rising constantly around us and are increasing our risk of suffering from a range of chronic health disorders. However, EMF exposes fetuses and babies to much higher health risks than adults.

If the existing standards are inadequate for adults, then they are certainly inadequate for fetuses, for babies and for young children for the following reasons:

1. Their bodies are forming rapidly and any damage to their DNA puts them at a much higher risk of developing morbid mutations with lifelong health consequences.

2. Their skulls and skeletons are much thinner and EMR penetrates much deeper into their brains and internal organs.

3. Their immune and nervous systems are still immature making them much more sensitive to electromagnetic radiation. Any adverse effect triggered within these systems may have immediate and far reaching consequences on their health including reduced immunity, increased susceptibility to infections, increased risk of childhood cancer and increased risk of behavioral disorders and developmental deficits.

Numerous studies have already shown that EMF results in increased risk to fetuses and pregnancies:

1. The 2012 Bioinitiative report states that there is evidence for fertility and reproduction effects and that the human sperm cells and their DNA are damaged.

2. Research has shown that exposure to radio frequency microwave electromagnetic radiation is associated with a higher risk of birth defects, and prenatal deaths

3. Studies have found that pregnant women exposed to electromagnetic radiation (EMR) are at a higher risk of miscarriages and late spontaneous abortions.

4. Scientists have concluded that fetal exposure to cellular phones leads to behavioral and neuro-physiological alterations that persist into adulthood.

5. Recent studies have indicated that exposure to electromagnetic radiation before and during pregnancy may expose the fetus and baby to ADHD, autism spectrum disorders (ASD), and increased incidence of various patterns of serious learning disabilities in young children (lower IQ).

6. Studies have shown that continued EMF exposure after birth might increase the harmful developmental disruption that occurred due to prenatal electromagnetic radiation exposure.

Pre and post-natal EMF protection strategy

The saying goes that an ounce of prevention is better than a pound of cure (especially in conditions for which there is no known cure). The way to prevent or at least reduce EMF health risks is to protect the sperm, fetus and baby from EMF exposure in every possible way. Here is an EMF protection action plan designed specifically for this purpose. This action plan requires using personal EMF protection accessories, such as cell phone radiation blocking cases, laptop anti-radiation pads, anti-radiation maternity clothing and blankets.

Protecting the sperm from electromagnetic radiation

Take these measures to reduce the risk of damage to sperm DNA as this may later express itself in the baby in all sorts of physiological and psychological disorders.

1. Wear electromagnetic radiation blocking boxer shorts or underwear.

2. Carry your cell phone in a cell-phone radiation blocking case.

3. Always try to put your laptop on a desk and not on your lap.

4. When using your laptop have an anti-radiation laptop shield between the laptop and your body (even if the laptop is on a desk).

5. If you do not have the anti-radiation laptop shield with you do not put the laptop on your lap.

Protecting the ovaries from electromagnetic radiation

Take these measures to reduce the risk of damage to ovaries and eggs that may later express itself in the baby in all sorts of physiological and psychological disorders.

1. Wear electromagnetic radiation blocking maternity clothing

2. Alternatively wear electromagnetic radiation blocking belly armor

3. Carry your cell phone in a radiation blocking case

4. When using your laptop use an anti-radiation shield between the laptop and your body.

Protecting the fetus from electromagnetic radiation

1. Wear electromagnetic radiation blocking maternity clothing

2. Alternatively wear electromagnetic radiation blocking belly armor

3. Carry your cell phone in a radiation blocking case

4. When using your laptop use an anti-radiation shield between the laptop and your body.

Protect pregnant mothers' blood cells from electromagnetic radiation

The quality of the mother's blood cells has a direct and immediate impact on the fetus. Since the blood flows throughout your body it is not enough to protect only your belly from electromagnetic radiation. You also need to protect the rest of your body from EMF exposure.

1. Protect your body from electromagnetic radiation by avoiding using cell-phones as much as possible. Also avoid Wi-Fi enabled devices including tablets, mini tablets, laptops and any PC that uses Wi-Fi to connect to the Internet.

2. If you must use your cell phone, always use an anti-radiation air tube headset or in emergencies use it in external speaker mode.

3. Carry your cell phone in a radiation blocking case

4. When using your laptop put an anti-radiation shield between the laptop and your body.

5. For extra protection when using a laptop use an EMF shielding blanket

Protecting the Baby from electromagnetic radiation

Babies should be kept away from any source of electromagnetic radiation including cell phones, Wi-Fi routers, DECT phones etc. These devices emit radiation even when not in use. To protect the newborn from EMR - 24/7. Follow these steps:

1. Get a reasonable quality EMF meter and a Dirty Electricity Meter. You may use a dual range (RF and LF) meter or a separate RF (radio frequency) meter and a LF (low frequency) EMF meter. These don't need to be professional grade only reasonably reliable.

2. Determine radiation levels in the baby's room: Measure LF and RF radiation levels. Put special emphasis on measuring radiation levels close to the baby's bed/crib/cot.

3. Measure dirty electricity levels in all electrical sockets in the baby's room.

4. RF radiation limits as recommended by the 2012 Bioinitiative report are: **0.3 nanowatts to 0.6 nanowatts per square centimeter (0.003 - 0.006 microwatt per square centimeter)** as a reasonable, precautionary action level for chronic exposure to pulsed RFR'.

5. **LF EMR limit recommended by the 2012 Bioinitiative report is 1 Milligauss.**

6. Dirty Electricity level recommended by Prof. Graham and Mr. David Stetzer is below 30 GS units and never above **50 GS units.**

7. If RF radiation levels in the baby's room are higher than the recommended levels, you need to take action to reduce the baby's EMR exposure. First, remove any source of wireless radiation from the baby's room (e.g. DECT cordless phones and their docking bases, Wi-Fi routers, computers and laptops connected via the home Wi-Fi or via a wireless broadband modem).

8. Re-measure levels of RF radiation in the baby's room if they are still too high you need to

identify the source outside the baby's room. If the source of RF EMR is your home wireless network, you need to reposition your Wi-Fi router as far away from the baby's room as possible. You then need to re-measure radiation levels. If these still prove too high, you must turn off the Wi-Fi and connect your PC or laptop to the router via a standard Ethernet cable (also called CAT 5e RJ45).

9. The source of RF radiation may be outside your apartment or house. Use an RF meter to identify the source of the radiation. It may be from a so-called "smart" meter. It may be from a nearby cell-phone tower. It may be coming from a neighbor's apartment. Some people have Wi-Fi routers in their apartments that are so powerful that expose their neighbors to significant amounts of electromagnetic radiation.

10. If the source of the radiation is a 'smart' meter connected to an external wall, refer to the section on Smart meters' self defense strategies and follow the instructions there. Also read the section on EMF RF shielding paints.

11. If the source of the RF radiation is a cell phone tower close by, the radiation may be penetrating the baby's room through one wall, two walls or even via the ceiling. In that case you may have to follow the procedure described in the section on Smart meters' self-defence strategies and EMF RF shielding paints. Protect all affected walls and if needed the ceiling as well if your measurements show that the radiation is also coming through your roof.

12. If the source of the RF radiation is a wireless router in a neighbor's apartment, you need to apply the procedure described in Smart meters' protection strategies to the wall(s) between your apartment and the room where your neighbor has positioned his wireless router.

13. If after taking all the above steps RF radiation levels are still too high in the baby's room you may consider hanging an anti-radiation shielding canopy over the baby's bed. The canopy looks like a big mosquito net used in tropical countries and you hang it from hooks inserted into the ceiling. You need to follow the manufacturer's instructions and make sure the canopy is well away from the baby's bed and does not dangle into the bed to prevent possible fatal choking hazards. The hooks should be able to support the weight of the

canopy.

Note: You may need to get a handyman to install the canopy for you if you are not a DIY person.

14. To reduce LF radiation exposure, move the baby's bed away from any source of electricity, including electrical wires and sockets, electrical power boxes (these may radiate via a wall and reach the baby) and electrical appliances. Note that refrigerators and air-conditioning systems in an adjoining room may radiate through the wall and reach the baby. Keep measuring until you position the baby in the safest place with the lowest level of LF radiation. If the results are still unsatisfactory you may need to move the baby to a different room.

15. If you find that your entire house has a high level of LF electromagnetic radiation this may prove to be a serious problem because unlike RF radiation that can be blocked with relative ease, LF radiation is very difficult and extremely expensive to deal with. You need to identify the external LF radiation source. If it is coming from a high tension power line running outside your house, you may need to consider relocation. If you are living in an apartment building the source of the LF radiation may also be the elevators' machine room or the central heating room or central air conditioning room. Blocking the LF radiation may be expensive as it requires tailor made metal alloy plates made and installed by a professional. In case you are renting you may consider relocating.

16. Refer to the section on "dirty electricity" and follow the instructions there. Basically you need to reduce the level to less than 50 GS (Graham Stetzer) units measured using a Dirty Electricity meter. You achieve this by installing one or two dirty electricity filters in the baby's room electrical sockets and perhaps one or two filters in electrical sockets in each of the adjoining rooms.

17. Many parents use baby monitoring or baby alarm systems. These systems are intended to monitor the baby when left in his/her bed without adult supervision and to make sure he is safe and sound. Some systems called baby cams also incorporate a video camera. Most baby monitoring and alarm systems use wireless RF technology. Some baby monitoring systems can be used in conjunction with a Smartphone by installing a special app on the

Smartphone. To reduce the baby's exposure to RF radiation you may consider installing a **wired** baby monitoring or baby alarm system instead of a wireless system. These systems serve the same function but instead of using wireless technology they transmit the data over wires. Some wired systems (using X10 and similar technologies) use existing household electrical wiring to avoid having to install wires along the walls. This technology increases levels of dirty electricity throughout your electrical network. Furthermore, installing dirty electricity filters in your house may possibly interfere with the operation of such wired systems. Avoid these problems by using a wired baby monitoring system that uses its own dedicated wires and not the houses' electrical network. These dedicated wires need to be installed along walls within plastic ducting.

Note: Installing any type of electrical wiring should be done only by a qualified electrician.

18. When you take your baby for a walk outside avoid power-lines, power-transformer stations, cell-phone towers and other microwave towers.

22 Children And Teenagers EMF Protection

Children EMF Protection

Children's immune system and nervous system are still developing and they are much more vulnerable to the morbid effects of electromagnetic radiation. Furthermore, children's skulls are much thinner than adult skulls and research has shown that cell phone radiation penetrates much deeper into children's brains than into adult brains. Children are growing and learning new things rapidly. Their minds are hungry for new information. The Internet is full of information, games and pictures and naturally they are drawn to it. Your challenge as a parent is to:

1. Make sure they connect to the Internet safely – using a PC connected to a router via an Ethernet cable with the Wi-Fi functionality disabled.

2. Make sure you protect them from exposure to inappropriate materials that the Internet is flooded with.

3. Make sure you protect them from contacting inappropriate or dangerous people online.

4. Make sure your children never disclose personal details online, including your credit card details!

To protect your children, follow the following steps:

1. Children should only be allowed to operate cell phones in emergencies. Cell phone manufacturers include warnings in the devices' manuals asking users to keep the phone 1.5 to 2.5 cm (about 0.6 - 1 inch) away from the head. Some scientists believe this is inadequate. But even if this were adequate for adults it is certainly inadequate for children for reasons explained above.

2. Children should not be allowed to play with mobile phones, tablets and other Wi-Fi enabled devices when the Wi-Fi is turned ON.

3. Do not use your cell-phone while standing close to children

4. Do not use Wi-Fi when children are in the house

5. Do not use your cell-phone with children in the car

6. When you take your children for a walk outside avoid power-lines, power-transformer stations, cell-phone towers and other microwave towers.

7. Set an example – minimize your own use of cell-phones and wireless devices, especially when your children are present and educate your kids about the inherent dangers of wireless technologies. You'd be surprised how quickly they learn and assimilate this information. Children have a much better access to their imagination than grownups and they have a much better ability at visualizing invisible electromagnetic fields than grownups.

Teenagers EMF Protection

Protecting teenagers from electromagnetic radiation is proving to be a very difficult task for several reasons:

1. Teenagers are very active socially. They have a strong need to communicate with their friends all the time. Teenagers seem to be glued to their Smartphones. They spend hours on Facebook, Google +, Gmail and all the other social networks.

2. Some teenagers spend much time downloading music and playing games online.

3. Teenagers are quick adopters of new technologies especially when it comes to wireless devices and the Internet.

4. Teenagers were born into the wireless information age. It seems natural to them and therefore hard to see mobile devices as a potential health hazard.

5. It can be difficult to tell teenagers what's good for them because they often think they know better.

So what can you do to protect your teenagers from EMF?

1. Lead by example – minimize your use of mobile technology and make a point of telling them about the inherent health risks of using this technology.

2. At home enforce a non-wireless wired only Internet connection. To do this effectively and fairly you will need to provide Ethernet cable connections running from the router to your kids' rooms. A professional can organize Ethernet cables neatly within plastic ducts running along walls and corners.

3. Provide your teenagers with wired telephones in their rooms so they can talk privately and maintain low EMR exposure.

4. Provide your teenagers with EMF protection accessories including air tube headsets, radiation redirecting Smartphone cases, radiation shielding phone cases, radiation blocking laptop pads, radiation blocking blankets.

23 Earthing

Since time immemorial man has lived in close contact with the earth, walking barefoot and sleeping on the ground. Wild animals still live this way. Modern man on the other hand, has lost touch with the earth in more ways than one. We wear shoes that have synthetic soles, our floors are covered with synthetic materials and we often live in high rise buildings far from the earth. We also live in a way that pollutes and creates imbalances in the environment with disregard to nature and mother earth. Our lifestyle and the conditions that we have created jeopardize our health in many ways. One of the most serious consequences of modern lifestyle is that we have become electrically insulated and disconnected from the earth.

Studies conducted since the 1960's have confirmed what Shamans and medicine men have known throughout the ages – that the earth has tremendous healing properties and that our well being depends on maintaining close contact with the earth. The surface of the earth is negatively charged and some scientists now think that the subtle flow of electrons from the earth via our feet and into our bodies may play a major role in controlling inflammatory processes and also in neutralizing free radicals throughout the body. Inflammatory processes are essential for fighting disease causing pathogens and for repairing damaged tissues throughout the body. However, if the body fails to control inflammation, then a state of chronic disease may ensue. Almost all diseases ending with an "itis" such as arthritis, tendonitis, bursitis, sinusitis, rhinitis, and colitis are inflammatory conditions. Many other diseases are also associated with a state of active inflammation. Scientists have found associations between inflammation and heart disease.

Technology and the chemical and electromagnetic pollution it creates all around us are producing significant amounts of free radicals. These are highly chemically reactive atoms, ions or molecules. Some free radicals cause cell damage and may have an adverse effect on human health. Free radicals may contribute to premature aging and development of disease such as cancer. Some scientists think that one of the natural mechanisms for controlling both inflammation and free radicals is the flow of negatively charged particles from the earth and into our bodies. Re-establishing this natural process may therefore have the potential to alleviate diverse disease conditions and improve overall health.

Clinton Ober, a retired cable TV executive, who was not a scientist by training has rediscovered these forgotten truths. Using his keen powers of observation and intuition he has come to the realization that many modern illnesses may be affected and/or aggravated by being electrically disconnected from the earth. Ideally we would all spend our lives walking barefoot in the park, on the beach and swimming in the ocean. However, since for most people this is not possible, Mr. Ober set out to develop various barefoot substitutes to enable people to stay connected to the earth without actually having to spend much time in nature. His innovations include earthed bed sheets, mats, hand and leg bands, recovery sleeping bags to name a few. These are all made from conductive materials and are connected via special wires and connectors to the house's electrical ground or to special rods inserted into the ground outside the house. Mr. Ober has collaborated with various scientists and they have shown in numerous studies that by using barefoot substitutes people have often regained their health and have overcome chronic long standing illnesses.

Another morbid aspect of modern lifestyle is that living and working close to power cables, electrical wiring and electrical devices induces substantial EMF induced voltage in our bodies. This unnatural voltage state may interfere with various electromagnetic aspects of our body and may weaken us and predispose us to disease. Earthing ourselves dramatically reduces EMF induced voltages by up to a factor of 1000. This is another mechanism by which earthing may help prevent disease and improve health and well-being.

24   DIY EMF Protection Or Using Professionals?

Things you can do yourself and things you can't

In these troubled financial times people do their best to reduce costs. One way to save money is DIY (Do It Yourself). Whether or not you should consider DIY depends on many factors including your technical skills, your time constraints and the severity of the situation. There are some things that are relatively easy to do by yourself provided you take the time to learn the basics. Other things should be done by professionals only. Here are some general guidelines for DIY versus using a professional:

1. **Electricity can kill or lead to serious bodily injury. Never attempt any type of electrical work yourself. Get a qualified electrician**.

2. Most low frequency (LF) radiation protection should be done by EMF professionals because LF protection usually requires considerable technical skills and may be quite expensive.

3. If you have poor technical skills and/or are very busy and/or are sick you should definitely use the services of an EMF consultant.

4. If you are considering buying a property and are concerned about EMF, you probably need to use the services of an EMF professional because of the significant investment and possible implications high EMF/EMR levels may have on the value of the property.

5. If you have reasonable technical skills and time on your hands, there are various EMF protection measures you can DIY. These include identifying potential EMF sources, conducting basic EMF measurements and applying basic EMF protection strategies. These include life style modifications, rearranging of living and work spaces, applying RF shielding paints, hanging RF shielding curtains and canopies, measuring dirty electrify and plugging in dirty electricity filters.

NOTE: Shielding paints usually require grounding plates and grounding connections. These should only be installed by a qualified electrician following manufacturer's instructions.

Getting an EMF professional

There are growing numbers of EMF protection professionals. Some specialize in Low Frequency (LF) protection, some in Radio Frequency (RF) protection and some do both. This is a relatively new field and often these people first got involved after having experienced the ill effects of EMF on their own health or the health of relatives and friends. I encourage you to seek these people's advice and guidance. You may have to pay them for a consultation but it may help you avoid mistakes and save you much money in the long run. Whenever you feel a problem may be beyond your knowledge or technical skills you should certainly seek professional help. An optimal approach may be to get a professional for an initial consultation and then ask the EMF professional to explain what you can do yourself and what you cannot do.

Getting a qualified electrician

As mentioned above EMF, EMR and electricity are intimately linked. At some point along your EMF protection journey you will need to use the services of an experienced and qualified electrician. It may be to test and repair your home's grounding, power-box or power-sockets. It may be to install grounding plates for your RF shielding paint. It may be to install or test the grounding for your earthing products. Electrical grounding especially in old houses is often faulty. The same applies to old power boxes. The entire wiring system in old houses has often been modified over the years resulting in a total hazardous mess. It needs to be checked methodically by a qualified electrician. Any work that involves electricity requires the help of a fully qualified and certified electrician.

CAUTION: Electricity can be very dangerous or even deadly and any sort of **electrical work should be done by qualified experienced electricians only.**

25 Affordable EMF Protection

Many people are experiencing financial uncertainty at present. Others may be living on a tight budget. Some of the EMF shielding and blocking techniques described in previous sections may be beyond your present means. But don't despair - there are all sorts of inexpensive EMF protection measures that you can use and still achieve good results in many cases.

There are steps you can take to reduce your EMF exposure without spending any money or spending very little. Of course nothing is absolutely free. You may have to give up well established habits, conveniences, opportunities and perhaps you may also need to devote more time when doing the same things that were so quick and easy using Wi-Fi and mobile technology. I know this is a significant stumbling block for many people on their path to EMF safety. For example, some people are finding it very difficult to give up their DECT phones because they are used to taking calls in bed or even in the bathtub. But think about it this way - it can be compared to the convenience of eating fast-food or take-away versus eating wholesome home-made freshly prepared food that requires more time and effort. In the long run, the time and money you save by eating fast food may be offset by the time you have to spend dealing with sickness and the money you may have to spend on doctors' bills, medications and hospitalizations not to mention the suffering and pain.

You can also look at it this way: The time you spend every day preparing healthy meals may be offset by years that will be added to your life. Similarly, since EMF/EMR exposure is cumulative any daily reduction in exposure will add up towards a safer, healthier and probably longer life. You can start with inexpensive EMF safety measures and apply additional more expensive measures when your financial situation allows.

Avoidance

We have discussed avoidance at length in a previous section. Avoidance is the most effective EMF protection method and it is also FREE although in some cases it may require making sacrifices that can be translated to considerable amounts of money (e.g. not accepting job offers that are associated with high EMR exposure). Here are some simple avoidance strategies that you can apply immediately at no cost or very cheaply:

1. Avoid using Wi-Fi. Disable the Wi-Fi functionality of your router and connect your computer or laptop to the router using Ethernet cables. Ethernet cables are inexpensive, the longer the cable you buy the cheaper it is per meter. However, if the cable is too long it tends to create a tangled mess. So try to buy the right length with a bit of length to spare in case you decide to rearrange your office later.

2. Avoid using Wi-Fi enabled devices. This means that you may have to avoid using your tablet and smartphone to connect to the Internet. Use your PC or laptop instead as described previously.

3. Avoid spending time, living or working in places that have high EMF/EMR levels. This may mean that you would need to relocate if you are living next to a substantial source of EMF that cannot be shielded against effectively.

4. Avoid walking close to LF and RF hazards such as high tension cables, power transformer stations, cell phone towers and other microwave telecommunication towers. Exercise is good for you. If your neighborhood is riddled with EMF hazards and you cannot move away, better stay indoors. Shield your home and get a treadmill for exercising. Of course treadmills have electric motors that generate LF electromagnetic radiation. So ideally you want to drive somewhere that is EMF safe, crime safe and has fresh air and do your walking or jogging there.

5. Avoid talking on your cell-phone or at least substantially reduce your air-time. That will save you time and money and reduce your EMF exposure.

6. If you must talk on your cell-phone use an air-tube headset. Avoid talking on the DECT

phone. Get rid of it - that won't cost you anything.

Affordable RF shielding techniques

RF shielding materials can be rather expensive. A typical RF shielding paint may cost more than ten dollars per square meter indoors and even more outdoors. RF shielding fabrics such as RF absorbing wallpaper, RF shielding transparent films for windows, RF shielding fabrics for curtains and partitions are even more expensive. However, there are several relatively inexpensive materials that can be used to achieve good RF shielding. They are not as good as the special purpose materials just mentioned but in some cases you may achieve very reasonable results.

REMEMBER: The only way to verify RF shielding quality is to measure RF radiation levels before and after applying your defensive measures.

Inexpensive general purpose materials with RF shielding properties

Here are several inexpensive general purpose materials that have <u>moderate</u> RF shielding properties and can be used as an additional or in some cases substitute for more expensive special purpose shielding materials:

1. **Metal insect screens**

   These can be used to protect windows, doors, external walls and roofs. They don't look so nice on internal walls but you can apply them on internal walls and then cover them with wallpaper or attractive fabrics. These screens are actually a wire mesh made of aluminium, galvanized iron, copper or stainless steel. The copper has the best EMR shielding properties but others will do. Buy several small samples first and test them at home on one window to see which works better for you. You can further improve RF shielding by using a double layer of the wire mesh. The more layers the better the shielding effect.

2. **Corrugated steel tile roofing**

   If you have tiles on your roof that need replacing you may consider redoing the entire roof with corrugated steel tile roofing. This type of roofing has much better RF shielding qualities than traditional tiles.

3. **Sandwich insulation panels under the roof**

    You may consider improving the insulation quality above your ceiling by incorporating sandwich insulating panels under the roof. These are usually made of several layers of polyurethane foam and steel/aluminum sheets. Make sure the panels incorporate steel and/or aluminum as this is what gives them their RF shielding qualities.

4. **Sandwich insulating panels in the walls**

    You may also consider improving the insulation quality of your walls by incorporating sandwich insulating panels in your walls. These are usually made of several layers of polyurethane foam and steel/aluminum sheets. Make sure the panels incorporate steel and/or aluminum as this is what gives them their RF shielding qualities.

5. **Multi-layer insulating materials**

    There is a wide range of multi-layer insulating materials that incorporate aluminum sheets and synthetic materials such as polyethylene foam. These have RF shielding properties and can also be applied under the roof, inside walls and partitions.

6. **Thermal aluminum foils**

    There is a wide range of thermal aluminum foils used for insulation. They are easier to work with than the multi-layer insulating materials mentioned above. They can also be used to improve insulation and provide RF shielding in your walls and under your roof.

7. **Mylar blankets**

    For EMF shielding smaller areas and when travelling you can also use Mylar blankets (also called thermal blankets, survival blankets, space blankets, first aid blankets, emergency blankets, or weather blankets). These have RF shielding properties that are much better than the aluminum foils you normally get in the supermarket because they are much thicker.

NOTE: Ordinary aluminum foils don't work well as shielding materials.

As you can see from the examples above there are many materials you can get at the hardware store and discount camping store that can serve as RF radiation shielding. After installing these materials, you need to re-measure radiation levels. If they are unsatisfactory you may need to do a bit more work. Often there are "cracks" in your EMF shielding in the corners of the walls and ceilings, around windows, around doors and so on. EMF can penetrate your defences through these cracks. EMF can also penetrate via gaps between adjacent aluminum sheets and panels so try to have them overlapping. By carefully measuring EMR around these areas you will be able to discover where the EMF is leaking through. You can then add more multi-layer thermal aluminum foil there or in some cases just use a bit of RF shielding paint only in the areas most difficult to shield. Shielding is both a science and an art so get creative!

Note: Infiltration and penetration of EMF/EMR via cracks, gaps and poorly applied shielding is especially true in the 5G millimeter bandwidth. Although to date (2021) there are no affordable commercially available RF meters for the millimeter bandwidth the rapid introduction of 5G and 'The Internet of Things' (IoT) will create a growing demand for such meters. Please refer to the following section on 5G EMF protection.

Affordable personal shielding

- Most people carry their cell-phones with them at all times. As recommended in previous sections, the cell phone should ideally be turned off or on airplane mode so it does not emit RF radiation that might penetrate your body. However, if that is not possible, and you don't want to invest in a cell-phone radiation blocking case you may still be able to block most of the radiation as follows: Get a little carry-bag. Pad the inside of the bag with multi-layer thermal aluminum foil or a thermal blanket. Make sure the thermal aluminum foil creates a barrier between your body and the cell-phone when the cell-phone is placed in the bag. The foil also needs to cover the bottom of the bag as EMR can leak through the bottom and reach your body. If the cell phone detects poor reception conditions, it may respond by increasing EMR output levels so you need to make sure that there is an opening in the insulation on the side of the bag facing away from you in such a way that the cell phone can easily transmit and receive signals. Get creative. Use your RF meter to test the results.

- If you are travelling and staying in a room with strong EMF/EMR you can use a thermal aluminum blanket to cover yourself at night and even during the day. This will keep you warm and reduce your EMF exposure.

Healthier and Cheaper

The saying "You get what you pay for" is often true but when it comes to reducing your exposure to EMF/EMR you get more for less! In other words, if you get a lower electric bill this is usually associated with lower EMF/EMR exposure. Consumption of electricity is in direct proportion to your usage of electrical and electronic devices. Each of these devices emits EMR and usually also introduces dirty electricity into your electrical network. Dirty electricity also produces EMR. Since electromagnetic radiation exposure is cumulative, any reduction in any type of EMF/EMR will reduce your overall exposure and lessen the burden and damage to your nervous system, immune system and every cell in your body.

One of the easiest and cost effective ways to reduce your EMR exposure is to consume less power. Here are a few simple ideas how you can reduce your power consumption and EMR exposure and save money:

1. In the winter, wear warm clothing indoors including thermal underwear, sweater, jacket, scarf and a warm hat. Wearing warm clothing indoors will allow you to lower the temperature inside the house by adjusting down your heating system's thermostat. Adjusting down the thermostat means that the system will work less frequently. This will reduce your electrical consumption and power bill and also reduce your overall EMR exposure. Of course, if you have a traditional fireplace this does not apply.

2. In the summer, wear light clothing indoors including a tee-shirt, shorts and sandals. Wearing light clothing indoors will allow you to raise the temperature inside the house by adjusting up the thermostat of your air-conditioning system. The system will then work less frequently. This will reduce your electrical consumption, lower your power bill and reduce your overall EMR exposure.

3. Use the dishwasher less frequently. Let the dirty dishes soak in soapy water and then brush and rinse them and let them dry. Some dish-washing liquids can be harsh on the hands resulting in dry skin so don't forget to use rubber gloves to protect your hands. Doing the dishes by hand will reduce your electrical consumption, lower your power bill and reduce your overall EMF exposure. If you must use your dishwasher, give the dishes a quick rinse

before putting them into the dishwasher and then choose the shortest cycle possible.

4. The best way to use solar power is using the sun to dry your laundry instead of using the dryer. This will reduce your electrical consumption, lower your power bill and reduce your overall EMF exposure. It may also improve air quality inside your house: Scientists have identified scores of hazardous air pollutants and known or probable carcinogens coming out of dryer vents. These include vapors from fabric softeners, fragrances and synthetic materials that contain residues of organic compounds including significant concentrations of acetaldehyde declared by International Agency for Research on Cancer (IARC) *"a probable or possible carcinogen in humans"* (i.e. may cause cancer).

5. Consider installing a solar water heating (SWH) system. These systems incorporate several innovations and technologies that have been used for many years in Australia, Austria, China, Cyprus, Greece, India, Israel, Japan and Turkey. They usually consist of a water tank, a solar collector and flexible water pipes. There is no need for water pumps or any electrical components as the water circulates naturally when its temperature rises as it flows through the solar collector. These systems save substantial amounts of electricity and lower EMR levels as they provide hot water without using electricity to heat the water. Of course, if you are using gas heaters to heat your water this does not apply. Also the efficiency of SWH systems depends on weather conditions, geographical latitude and available sunshine so installing them in the North Pole may not be a good idea.

26 '5G' EMF Protection

Generally, the same principles and methods described in previous chapters also apply to 5G EMF/EMR detection and protection. However, there are several aspects of 5G rollout and high frequency band 5G ('millimeter waves') that require special consideration.

As discussed in previous chapters, the first step in mitigating EMR is measuring it. You need to know EMR exposure sources and levels you are dealing with. Most good EMF RF meters cover the entire range of 3G and 4G frequencies, as well as low and middle 5G frequency bands, and are typically capable of measuring up to 8 Ghz. However, existing meters do not cover the 5G millimeter wave bands. Meters for measuring these bands are not commercially available to date (January 2021) and are only used by some professionals and scientists. As a matter of fact, most EMF 'consultants' cannot afford these specialized devices. These meters may also require more technical understanding and special antennas.

The good news is that at least inside your home you could be relatively safe from high frequency millimeter wave 5G if you follow EMF protection advice given in previous chapters and specific advice given in this chapter. As a matter of fact, there are many actions that you can take right now and in the near future to significantly decrease your exposure to 5G EMR, including high band 5G frequencies (millimeter waves) as follows:

1. As mentioned in previous chapters one of the most effective methods to protect yourself is to **keep a safe distance from sources of RF EMF.** In urban areas, "small cell" 5G antennas may appear in the near future next to your house or apartment, on utility poles, lamp posts etc. This may increase EMR energy density by a factor of thousands! Electro Hypersensitive people (EHS) are already being forced to move out of cities to the countryside and many more people may develop EHS and be forced to move away from urban areas.

2. However, for many people moving away may not be an option. In this case, **try to live as far as possible from any antennas**. 5G has a short range and is obstructed easily by physical objects and therefore the back part of a house or building (away from the street) may be much safer than the front part.

3. Reduce the risk by not living or working where you have a direct line of sight to a 4G/5G antenna. In other words, **these antennas should not be visible from any of your windows,** working and living spaces.

4. High frequency band 5G (millimeter waves) have a much shorter wavelength than 4G (centimeter waves). The good news is that millimeter waves are obstructed and blocked by physical and living objects (e.g. walls, trees). However, the bad news is that **they are able to penetrate your home through much smaller gaps between walls, windows and doors, roofs and walls and between elements of EMF blocking materials that are not continuous or overlapping** (e.g. EMF blocking paint, EMF blocking wallpaper, EMF blocking curtains, EMF blocking transparencies etc.). You will need to be very meticulous when installing EMF blocking materials. You may need to improve the continuity of EMF blocking materials using high conductivity EMF shielding tapes.
CAUTION: EMF shielding tapes can conduct electricity and become a safety hazard if installed in close proximity to electric sockets, wiring or appliances. Seek the assistance of an EMF specialist and electrician.

5. RF EMF protective materials work by incorporating RF EMF blocking particles or fibers into the material. The density of the particles or fibers needs to be much higher to block 5G millimeter waves because of their much smaller wavelength that allows them to 'sneak in' through the mesh. You may need to contact the manufacturers and verify that the products are effective for protecting against 5G EMF.

6. If you have already fortified your house and office using RF EMF protective materials (such as EMF blocking paint, wallpaper, curtains, transparencies, canopies, pads etc.) you may need to contact the manufacturers and verify that the products are also effective for protecting against 5G EMF.

7. If you go outside wearing RF EMF protective clothing and hats you may need to contact the manufacturers and verify that the products are also effective for protecting against 5G EMF.

8. **Remove the 'Internet of Things' (IoT) from your home and from your life**. Do not buy any devices that have IoT functionality. You may be able to get a technician to disable the IoT functionality on some devices (e.g. refrigerators). Do not buy any consumer products that have IoT sensors or remove them if you can (e.g. from packaged or canned products that are stored in the fridge).

9. **Connect all home devices to the router using ethernet cables and disable the Wi-Fi functionality of any router in your home**. Most routers have a Wi-Fi on/off button that allows you to do it easily. Do not buy or install a router that does not come with such a button.

10. **Connect to your Internet service provider using fiber optic or copper cables only**. Refuse any offer to be connected to the internet or other services using 5G instead of cable or fiber optic.

11. Do not buy and install light fixtures that transmit 5G frequencies.

12. Minimize the use of cell phones and Wi-Fi routers indoors. This is discussed in previous chapters but is even more crucial if the devices have 5G functionality. For example, 5G cell phones and routers will typically emit much stronger EMR levels to overcome 5G's difficulty in penetrating walls and doors.

13. 5G millimeter radiation coming from satellites is also a source of concern and may require giving more thought to EMF RF protecting materials used in roofs and walls and types of insulation incorporated in roofs and walls.

27 Green Is Not Always EMF Clean

The energy crisis and global warming has given rise to a host of green technologies. Most people probably agree that we need to try to reduce power consumption in order to reduce greenhouse emissions, slow down global warming and prevent the creation of destructive weather patterns. As explained in previous sections reducing power consumption may also help decrease levels of EMR in the environment and in our homes. A host of technologies have been developed to help save energy and reduce power consumption. Overall these technologies are a positive step in the right direction. However, it needs to be pointed out that some of these technologies may contribute to significant increases in EMR exposure and associated health risks. I am sure the people who developed them and introduced them were not aware of some of these possible consequences. Let's just look at a few examples:

1. Fluorescent lamps and compact fluorescent lamps (CFLs) are being introduced on a very large scale. These lamps are much more energy efficient than traditional incandescent lamps. However, Fluorescent lamps and CFLs generate much higher LF EMR than incandescent lamps and they also generate considerable levels of dirty electricity. Most older fluorescent lamps and many (but not all) CFLs contain mercury and if broken accidentally or disposed of incorrectly may release mercury into the environment.

2. There are several types of solar power systems that use solar panels made from arrays of photo-voltaic cells to generate electricity. In principle these systems are designed to use a renewable source of energy (solar) instead of burning fossil fuels. Some solar power systems work off the grid and some are connected to the grid. The ones that work off the grid are designed to provide electrical power in remote locations. The ones that are connected to the grid are designed to generate power that goes back into the grid in exchange for credit that is later deducted from your electricity bill. This is all

good because it reduces burning of fossil fuels and helps to reduce global warming. A potential EMF issue with these systems results from the fact that solar panels generate DC voltage that fluctuates with the sunlight's intensity. However, in order to feed the generated power into the grid or use it to power electrical appliances it needs to be converted to a specific fixed AC voltage. This is done using electrical components called inverters. Inverters tend to generate substantial levels of LF EMR that may be hundreds of times greater than the upper safety limit of 1 mG recommended by the 2012 Bioinitiative Report. In order to overcome this problem, the inverters should be positioned well away from living and work areas.

3. Hybrid and Electric Vehicles are discussed in more detail in the section on EMF in cars. These were designed to reduce air pollution in urban areas and also contribute to the fight against global warming by reducing the usage of fossil fuels. However, both Hybrid and electric cars generate much higher levels of EMF/EMR than traditional cars.

Figure 27.1 High EMF 'Green Technologies'

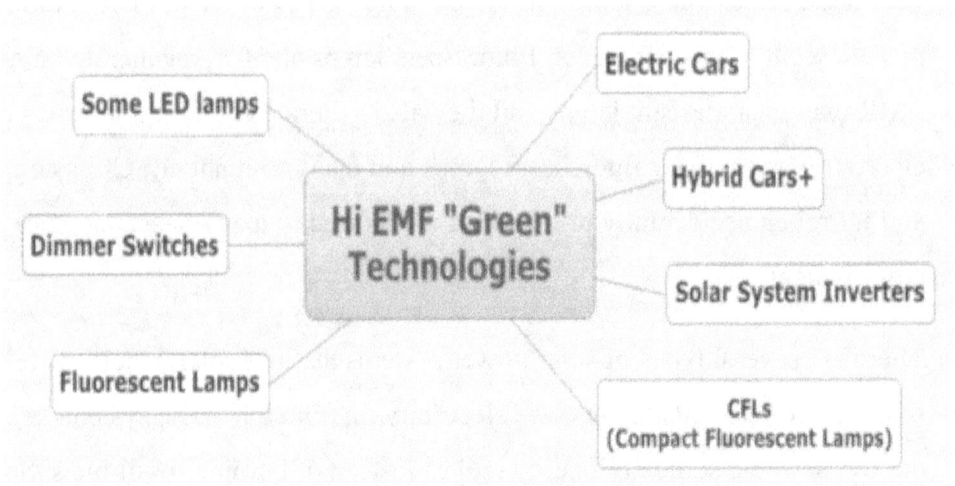

28 . Holistic & Alternative EMF Protection Methods

A holistic approach to health and medicine focuses on the person as a whole and not just on the disease and its symptoms as conventional medicine often tends to do. Holistic medicine aims at addressing all aspects of the mind-body in order to bring them into balance and harmony and maximize the person's innate healing powers. Holistic medicine is a very important and interesting area of health and wellbeing and I encourage you to read and learn more about it. Holistic approach to health and medicine is beyond the scope of this book yet I feel that several issues need addressing as there seems to be some confusion about them.

Some natural remedies and herbal extracts have been shown in studies to assist in alleviating the effects of ionizing radioactive radiation. There are various herbal remedies, homeopathic remedies and other supplements that are claimed to reduce, mitigate or neutralize effects of non-ionizing electromagnetic radiation. Obviously, I have not researched or evaluated most of these products. However, to date I have not seen any scientific evidence to substantiate any of the claims made about the ability of these products to counteract the effect of non-ionizing electromagnetic radiation.

I do believe that there are many herbs, herbal formulations, plant extracts and other supplements that may provide immense benefits in maintaining or even restoring health. Some natural and traditional remedies have been examined in numerous scientific studies and have been shown to have greater efficacy than conventional drugs with much lower toxicity and associated side effects. HOWEVER, you should ALWAYS seek the help and supervision of a health care provider and NEVER self-prescribe any of these herbal and other supplements.

There are various biofeedback systems, pendants, medallions, necklaces, disks, microchips and stones that are claimed to reduce, mitigate or neutralize electromagnetic radiation or its effects on the body. The advertisements talking about these products often refer to research that is supposed to back these claims. Obviously, I have not researched or tested most of them nor do I intend to do so. However, all products that I have researched or tested did not seem to have ANY measurable effect on EMF/EMR exposure levels or on measurable physiological parameters. The evidence supplied by some manufacturers does not satisfy the requirements of gold standard scientific investigation to say the least. Radio Frequency (RF) engineering is a very complex field. Because of the complexity and infinite variability of tests that can be conducted it is not easy to design a robust and reliable study.

Now here is the problem: Technologically naive people may easily be misled into believing a particular gadget will solve all their EMF exposure problems. Sadly, this is not the case. EMF radiation pollution is one of the most serious health problems of our time and it cannot be solved with a wave of a magic wand or a magic pendant. I wish it were – because I have always loved technology and innovation and still do. However, my electro hypersensitivity has forced me to take a second look at life style and reassess the benefit versus potential harm of many of the gadgets we have come to rely upon.

A story to illustrate the point. A friend's office was relocated right next to a telecommunication relay station. All of sudden she found herself looking through the window at a huge telecommunication tower with a multitude of antennas of all shapes and sizes. As you may have expected RF radiation levels there were quite high. I couldn't help noticing a little sticker taped to the top corner of my friend's computer screen. It was a nice colorful sticker that looked like some sort of new age meditation "Yantra". My friend had bought it at a new age store. The lady at the store explained that by gazing frequently at this special drawing, our subconscious mind is programmed to protect itself and the whole body from electromagnetic radiation.

Now don't get me wrong. I do believe the "placebo effect" may influence health, healing and disease. Research has shown that patients given sham sugar pills have often recovered from very serious medical conditions because they believed the pills were actually a new and very effective medicine. The Holy Bible also talks about the power of faith and its ability to make miracles happen. However, don't you think it would be wiser to first take EMF protection steps that have been technologically and scientifically tested and proven?

REFERENCES

- Parliamentary Assembly Council of Europe (2011). Resolution on the potential dangers of electromagnetic fields and their effect on the environment (Resolution 1815), 2014, from http://assembly.coe.int/Mainf.asp?link=/Documents/AdoptedText/ta11/ERES1815.htm

- Bioinitiative Report (2012). THE BIOINITIATIVE REPORT 2012 - A Rationale for Biologically-based Public Exposure Standards for Electromagnetic Fields (ELF and RF), 2014, http://www.bioinitiative.org/

- WHO (2005). Electromagnetic fields and public health - Electromagnetic Hypersensitivity Retrieved 2014, from http://www.who.int/peh-emf/publications/facts/fs296/en/

- Hillert, L., N Berglind, Arnetz, B., & Bellander, T. (2002). Prevalence of self-reported hypersensitivity to electric or magnetic fields in a population-based questionnaire survey. Scand J Work Environ Health, 28 (1(1)), 33-41.

- Roosli, M., Moser, M., Baldinini, Y., Meier, M., & Braun-Fahrlander., C. (2004). Symptoms of ill health ascribed to electromagnetic field exposure--a questionnaire survey. Int J Hyg Environ Health, 207 (2), 141-150.

AFTERWORD

It is time to say goodbye. I hope you have enjoyed reading this book. I hope this book will help you deal with EMF challenges in your life. This book although small in size contains a substantial amount of information. You may benefit by going over it again and again until you have digested all the information well. You may also refer to the book whenever a new EMF issue appears in your life.

EMF and EMR will be going away any time soon. On the contrary, EMF health hazards are growing daily, becoming more diverse, powerful and morbid. Anyone interested in regaining or maintaining his/her health and the health of loved ones needs to keep up to date and maintain vigilance. I believe that you do not have to be a scientist or an engineer to protect yourself effectively against Electromagnetic Fields (EMF) and electromagnetic radiation (EMR). I believe that after having read this book you are in a better position to take action to protect yourself from EMFs. Please follow the procedures and guidelines described in this book when measuring electromagnetic radiation levels, analyzing the results and formulating your EMF self-defence strategies. Make a detailed well-structured plan of action and stick to it. Never give up.

There are growing numbers of EMF protection professionals. Some specialize in Low Frequency protection (LF) and some in Radio Frequency (RF) protection and some in both. This is a relatively new field and often these people first got involved after having experienced the ill effects of EMF on their own health or the health of relatives and friends. I encourage you to seek these people's advice and help whenever you feel a problem may be beyond your knowledge or technical skills. At some point along your EMF protection journey you will need to use the services of an experienced and qualified electrician. It may be to test and repair your home's grounding, power-box or power-sockets. It may be to install grounding plates for your RF shielding paint. It may be to install or test the grounding for your earthing products. Electrical grounding especially in old houses may be faulty and hazardous. The same applies to old power boxes. The entire wiring systems in old houses have often been modified several times by various people resulting in a total dangerous and ugly mess and needs to be checked methodically by a qualified electrician.

REMEMBER: Electricity can be very dangerous or even deadly and any sort of electrical work should be done by qualified experienced electricians only.

I have done my best to make this book clear, concise, practical and actionable. I am not a professional writer so I must apologize in advance if this book fails to meet your perfectly justified literary and grammatical standards. If you have any comments, feedback, or suggestions on how I can improve this book in any way please do not hesitate to email me and I will do my best to improve this book and make it better and more useful in any way possible.

Stay EMF safe and NEVER give up!

Dr. Jonathan Halpern, PhD

ABOUT THE AUTHOR

Jonathan Halpern, PhD (Health Sciences), MSc (TCM), BSc (Engineering) areas of interest include Electromagnetic Fields and Health, Health Sciences, Alternative & Complementary Medicine and Public Health.

Jonathan first became aware of the adverse effects that Electromagnetic Radiation (EMR) has on health when he started using his first cell phone and discovered he was Electro Hypersensitive (EHS) long before the syndrome became widely recognized. Jonathan's electro-hypersensitivity triggered a keen interest in the body's electromagnetic fields and their role in health and disease.

Jonathan's research over the years has made him realize that many aspects of plant, animal and human life depend on a fine balance between positive and negative electrical charges, fine-tuned subtle electromagnetic fields and a constant electromagnetic flow on the cellular, tissue and systemic levels. Jonathan has also found that our body's electromagnetic balance is severely compromised as a result of the proliferation of wireless technology and electricity.

Electromagnetic Radiation Survival Guide - Step by Step Solutions

https://www.amazon.com/dp/B00HKMCQEY

Electromagnetic Radiation Survival Guide is a practical and actionable step by step , complete and up to date EMF/EMR detection and protection guide and reference manual. It covers the most important EMF/EMR issues including 5G, cell phone & telecommunication towers, smart meters, cell phones, tablets, laptops, Wi-Fi, Blue-tooth, hi voltage electrical cables, electrical appliances and wiring.

The proliferation of electrical power and wireless technology has caused a massive increase in electromagnetic fields (EMF) in our environment. There is now substantial scientific evidence that Electromagnetic Radiation (EMR) exposure well below existing safety standards may cause a range of bio-effects that increase the risk of serious diseases including cancer, neuro-degenerative disorders, sleep disorders and behavioral disorders.

 Indeed EMF has become one of the greatest health hazards of our times. The time to protect ourselves against electromagnetic radiation is NOW.

Healthy Smoothie Recipes: How to make Smoothies for Diet, Weight loss, Detox & Energy

https://www.amazon.com/dp/B01E3CJBBE

Quick, easy and flexible smoothies for boosting and balancing nutrition while accommodating a busy lifestyle based on the principles of modern nutrition science, alternative and complementary medicine and traditional medicine. For all seasons, individual needs, preferences and conditions.

This book is for you if you want to Improve your well-being, feel lighter and energized, diet easier and save time and money.The recipes are super healthy, low calorie, detoxing, energizing, quick, easy, tasty and balanced.

The book includes detailed information on the ingredients, and provides essential information for making balanced smoothies, adapting smoothies to needs, seasons and diets.

Zooock crashes on Earth : An alien and a boy go on an amazing adventure (for ages 9 -13)

https://www.amazon.com/dp/B08PDZ9SSQ

Kids who love adventures, aliens, space, planets, spacecraft and spaceships, flying drones, science and technology, computers and telescopes - will love this fun, relevant and action-packed story about 10-year old Luke Smith and his new friend the alien Zooock from Planet Gooock whose spacecraft crashed on Earth. Together they go on amazing adventures as Luke tries to help Zooock get back home and avoid being captured by a greedy and powerful tycoon who wants to get his hands on advanced alien technologies and doesn't hesitate to use his cunning henchman to achieve his goals. However, in the end, great friendship, courage and an ability to learn, improvise and take risks overcome all challenges. The story is entertaining, funny, exciting and educational with snippets of interesting information on astronomy, telescopes, drones, health and wellbeing, family life and more.

www.ingramcontent.com/pod-product-compliance
Lightning Source LLC
Chambersburg PA
CBHW081435250726
48662CB00009B/2803

9 798596 671865